MENTAL HEALTH FOR MILLENNIALS

Vol 6

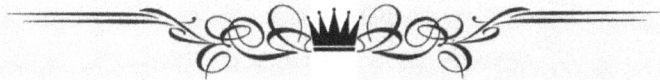

On 'Hope and Inclusion'

Series Editors

Dr. Niall MacGiolla Bhuí
Dr. Phil Noone

Volume Editor Giselle Marrinan M.Sc.

This Series is peer reviewed.

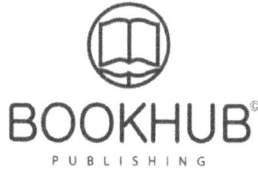

BOOKHUB©
PUBLISHING

Published by Book Hub Publishing, an Independent Publishing House with Offices in Athenry, Galway and Limerick, Ireland.
Book 6 in the TheDocCheck.Com 'Millennials' Series

This Series is sponsored by Relational Research and Consulting Ltd.

www.bookhubpublishing.com
www.thedoccheck.com
www.dissertationdoctorsclinic.com

@BookHubPublish @ThesisClinic

Dr. Niall MacGiolla Bhuí and Dr. Phil Noone are Series Editors (2017-2023).
Giselle Marrinan, M.Sc. is Co-Editor on this collection of chapters.

Cover photography by Niall MacGiolla Bhuí (photographs taken on location in Blackrock, Galway, Ireland)

ISBN: 978-1-7391012-5-1

Our books are printed on forestry sustainable paper. Viva la forests!

About the Clinic Series

The purpose of this DocCheck.Com Mental Health for Millennials Series is to encourage us all to read current material on various themes related to millennial life that is grounded in experience, with a backdrop in theory, written in a style that is fully accessible, interesting and genuinely meaningful to the daily experiences of us all. This is book six of our series with one more book scheduled to follow (2017-2023). We included the guest chapters in this book because we all believe the themes of hope and inclusion, in the context of millennials, deserves greater attention. Our aspiration is that these books will facilitate readers to understand in a little more detail, the dynamics of millennial life as it is experienced, through providing frameworks for conceptualisation and practice.

This series is designed to be useful for: 1) the individual looking to enhance their knowledge about millennials and mental health and wellness 2) the interested professional who does not want to read purely theoretical material. And, make no mistake; lives are complex for millennials. The age of the Internet and 'wearable technologies' presents many challenges - some foreseen but, oh so many, not so. In all of this, millennials are trying to make sense of themselves and their lives and we are trying to make sense of them (that's the older contributors in this book. We've also included several chapters written by millennials for balance).

The series itself is intended, therefore, not just to be 'books to read' but also as reference guides. Feel free to dip in and out of whatever chapter takes your fancy. We're not precious about individual chapter ownership and include essays on a range of topics. Happy reading.

Dr. Niall MacGiolla Bhuí

Table of Contents

CREATIVE WRITING

Looking Back to Look Forward: Challenging 'Cafocracy Conversation' and Advocating a Culture of Hope

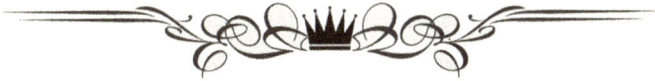

Dr. Niall MacGiolla Bhuí

"Lá Fhéile Pádraig sona daoibh - Happy St Patrick's Day to you."

Introduction

In volumes 1-5 of this book series, I've championed the millennial cohort. In this volume, I want to challenge them. Millennials have many wonderful characteristics but millennials can be racist - just like any other generation. This is not something I state lightly, but it is a worrying emerging theme in the published research and across social media and, later in this chapter, I'll cite some of the more interesting studies that have grabbed my attention.

I engage with the concept of racism in the context of my own experiences as a Generation X youthful university student over the

1

duration of my undergraduate and postgraduate degrees undertaken in Ireland in the 1980s and 1990s. During this period, I regularly ventured from Galway in the west of Ireland over to London in the UK to work and live.[1] The chapter then moves to commenting on millennial discourse around this theme and asks whether millennials exist in a more *inclusive* and *hopeful* environment than was the case when I was the same age category – just at a different point in time.

Further, it asks whether millennials may be said to be a more *informed* generation on matters of racism and race relations than we were at their same age points (in our 20s and 30s). Of course, these are my own views on lived experiences abroad and they don't claim to be representative of all the Irish living and working in London or the UK more generally where many of my friends had, and continue to have, a 'grand old time'.

Let's commence by offering a definition of racism. In Ireland, the National Consultative Committee on Racism and Interculturalism (NCCRI) defines racism as:

> *"A specific form of discrimination faced by minority ethnic groups based on the false belief that some 'races' are in essence superior to others because of different skin colour, nationality, ethnic or cultural background".*

Statistics in Context

Ah. Statistics. Between 1846 and 1855, over 300,000 Irish emigrated to Britain. At the time of writing this chapter, there are some 600,000 people living in the UK who declare themselves as Irish, with

---

[1] Generation X covers people born from 1965 through 1980.

200,000 Irish working in the NHS (Llyod, 2022). Skyrocketing unemployment in Ireland in the 1980s when I was studying at university, triggered a decade of emigration with many of my peers emigrating to the UK to start new lives, all too many of them never to return to Ireland to work, live and raise their families. This has been the history of the Irish. In the 1990s, our now infamous 'Celtic Tiger' economy attracted, for the first time, swathes of foreign-born immigrants and, happily, some of our emigrants returned to us. This changed, once again, post 2008 after the global financial crisis where we, once again, returned to emigration to many countries including the UK. Only last month, a good friend of mine emigrated to London with his child. 'The times they repeat themselves'.

A Casual Ignorance of the Irish

And yet, despite centuries of back and forth to the UK, there remains, with our neighbours across the Irish sea, what I might describe as a 'casual ignorance' of many things 'Ireland' and 'Irish'. There seems to be a habit of downgrading the significance of *Irishness* not just in the minds and attitudes of the so-called British "chumocracy" as noted by Bagehot (2018). This plays out in the public schools and their Oxford/Cambridge-educated elite, but also filters down to each strata of British society within organisations, agencies and institutions. In fact, I've often rather surreptitiously tuned in to what I'll coin as a 'cafocracy conversation' over a mug of (English) tea sitting in a roadside café in north London. By this, I mean the pseudo-democratic conversations that are often the preserve of such environments where 'Paddys' and 'Pakkis' are the subject of some mirth amongst the 'real English'.

And this attitude extends itself into the academic and research worlds. Indeed, Miles (1982) posed the question thirty years ago, to what extent would developing an Irish dimension involve an important reformulation of concepts of racism built around skin colour rather than other (real, imagined) phenotypical and cultural characteristics? (Cited in Hickman & Ryan, 2020).

The Cause of Irishness and Racism

The cause of 'Irishness' can best be approached via a careful examination through a historical lens. This, unfortunately, speaks to dominant colonial relations where we Irish have, for centuries, been seen as a potential reserve army of labour for mainland Britain. Ironically, many commentators suggest that Irish labour will, once again, prop up specific sectors of the British economy. True, the various Common Travel Area agreements, on the surface, granted the Irish in Britain a welcome level of access and entitlement over the years, but the anti-terrorist legislation from the 1970s to 1990s let us very clearly witness the fragile ground on which Irish rights and a sense of 'belonging' hung precariously (Hickman & Ryan, 2020).

Thankfully, racism is now a dominant theme across news channels and the ubiquitous social media, giving me hope for a more truly inclusive global society where older, entrenched attitudes might eventually evaporate into the ether. Racism and racist attitudes are actively challenged at every point. It might seem extraordinary but Hickman & Ryan (2020) note how even though the Irish remain one of the largest migrant groups to the UK, they have been overlooked in much research.

So, here's what I think. It is deeply ironic to all of us Irish that Ireland is, in fact, largely invisible (of course, not exclusively) to England

and the English in a way Britain/England can never be invisible to Ireland. We simply do not matter in the greater scheme of things to the mainland. We are those annoying, noisy neighbours across the water.[2] We are the little brother. No, we're just one of the little irksome brothers scattered around the world. Occasionally, we send the mainland a millennial or gen z soccer wunderkid to play in their Premier League...And the fans are thankful. But is there still an institutional *racist* attitude towards the Irish?

Our Experience as Irish in London

Before I answer that specific question, I want to return to life in the 1980s when a group of us Irish university students first arrived into central London armed with our Walkmans, backpacks and London AZ books and fanned out on the busy underground system looking for accommodation and summer work. Being an English Literature student, I marvelled at the poetry that hung on the Tube carriages. What I didn't admire was the almost immediate and frequent jibes of 'Hello Paddy", "Alright Seamus?" and, as it was the 1980s, "Are you in the IRA Paddy and do we need to sit well away from you?"[3]

I didn't admire being spat on and told to "Fuck off back to the bogs" outside concerts in Finsbury Park or the Electric Ballroom in Camden. I did not like the casual way we Irish were frequently stopped and

---

[2] Britain continues, somehow, to delight in attempting to steal our Irish glory; our musicians, sportspersons, our poets, dramatists and novelists are consistently 'British' when they win awards.

[3] The Birmingham Pub Bombings were carried out by the IRA in November 1974 in central Birmingham killing 21 people. The Prevention of Terrorism Act was passed by parliament a few days later. Thus, these remained in the public consciousness just over a decade later.

searched by police officers in central London simply because we were in well-known Irish areas. I quickly lost count of the number of times we Irish were casually picked out from the crowds in Speaker's Corner and searched. We had come from ordinary homes in the mid-west and west of Ireland; housing estates, farms, semi-detached and detached homes on streets. This was not in our everyday lexicon.

Several of us Arts and Science students ended up in North London in areas such as Camden Town, Kentish Town and Archway where the Irish had a long and established history living and working. 'The craic was good in Cricklewood'…But, our time there was not one without its challenges. Looking back now, I see these times as ones where profound racism against the Irish and being stereotyped into only certain job roles was the norm rather than the exception. We lived this on a daily basis and it filled me with frustration as I had an English mother and Irish father and I, naively, expected better. It's so different to what I see with millennials and gen z students in London now and it makes me wonder, how different is life for the generations behind me?

Perhaps it's about that word *expectation*. 'Back in the day' we did not have massive expectations as we heard so many negative stories from our peers. We read newspaper reports, we studied sociological and political science and we listened to radio and watched both Irish and English TV programmes. But we felt we had one crucial thing in our collective and individual armouries – we were university students. We were educated, or at least we were 'in education' and would be respected for this. Our experience away from our homes – Ireland – Mayo, Galway, Roscommon, Sligo, Donegal and Clare would surely be qualitatively different than that of generations before us.

The Contemporary Experience of being Irish in the UK

We are now inundated with coverage of the Brexit negotiations and the(ir) decision 'to leave', and, more recently, (again!) the complexities of the Northern Ireland border and issues of sovereignty. Clearly, the history and nuance of British–Irish relations remains complex and not very well understood by all-too-many influential politicians. The recent death of the British Monarch, Queen Elizabeth 11, has occasioned much patriotism and jingoism again. But is there room for hope? Are millennials and gen z living in a more inclusive time than we older observers did at their ages and is this inclusivity a composite of the millennial mindset?

The 2016 EU Referendum has found Britain actively preparing to leave the EU and former accepted migrant privileges are now, at best, uncertain. Rzepnikowska (2018) notes the increasing volume of attacks on white migrants where accent and language substitute for skin colour. This is worrying for the Irish and, particularly, our millennial and gen z populations. And yet, our youthful Irish migrants continue to fill labour market vacancies, often in roles English workers do not want to take up. They are needed. In some sectors.

Millennials and Racism

The label millennial refers to those born after 1980 – the first generation to come of age in the new millennium. In a recent European Broadcasting Union's massive 'Generation What' survey (2016) including eighteen countries, only 23% of 16-25 year olds in the Irish cohort thought they would *not* do as well as their parents. Overall, happiness (65%) was ranked the single most important factor in a successful life, beating out having a family, a job or money (we dedicated volume 4 of this book series to the theme of happiness). Interestingly, almost half (49%) were confident they would *do better* and 71% of Irish young people reported being *optimistic* about what comes next. But what does come next?

In the context of this chapter, I was disappointed with the European Broadcasting Union's report (2016) that only 60% of Irish respondents agreed *"immigration makes for stronger cultures"* as a figure of 40% either not agreeing or being unsure seems way too high for such a supposedly enlightened generation. That is not, of course, to argue that millennials are racist per se, rather it notes a reluctance to accept and promote travel, work, lived life in another country – presumably because such people are *different*. And, such attitudes can creep ever so slowly to racist ideologies if not actively challenged.

This is mentioned in that, in global terms, it is argued that millennials "appear more sensitive to institutional discrimination than their older peers" (Davis, 2019). A point confirmed in an earlier (2009) Pew Research survey, where *younger* (my emphasis) millennials are reported as being more receptive to immigrants than are their elders with 58% stating immigrants strengthen the country. Worryingly, when we look to the older millennials, just 43% agree. So, is the problem with older millennials, those in the 35 to 40 age group?

DeSante and Smith (2020) caution that millennials "are not relying on "older" versions of racial animus or explanations of persistent racial disparities, but instead employ a new set of racial logics - a mix of colourblind racial ideology and diversity ideology. Both allow millennials to appear to be more racially progressive because, on the surface, they claim "to not see race" while also appreciating racial diversity. Nonetheless, these ostensible humanist views are mitigated by what we see as a set of countervailing forces." A powerful observation.

Millennials have frequently been described as an entitled, narcissistic, app-obsessed, participation-trophy generation. I would argue that there is an element of truth in this (I always smile at the Apple watch phenomenon of sending 'reward' notifications on very basic exercise completion etc) but also that millennials have occupied the forefront of some of the key issues of the 21st century, and included in this is questioning racial and economic inequality.

I see this in my daily work at my Dissertation Clinic, where I regularly supervise millennial clients on these themes. Indeed, the term 'post racial' is now in use to speak to the levels of awareness of millennials around race issues. And yet, there is this niggling 'rainbow of discrimination' (Gaddis, 2021) that worries me. This needs to be challenged at every point and none of us should leave it to others to take up the mantle. Let's all be active.

This brighter and more hopeful future must be one where racism is challenged and where dialogue takes centre stage in attempting to uncover, understand and appreciate the cultural differences between nation states and the people who move back and forth between them. Ironically, we felt in the 1980s that it would become easier to seamlessly move and work between and within countries with an absence of racist undertones in expressing our Irish identity, particularly with our closest neighbour in their capital city in a spirit of inclusivity. Hope is, indeed, that most precious of things…As we might say to our neighbours on our most auspicious of days,

"Lá Fhéile Pádraig sona daoibh - Happy St Patrick's Day to you."

References

Bagehot. (2018). *The Times*. Downloaded on 8th May 2022 at: https://www.economist.com/britain/2018/12/22/the-elite-that-failed. [Google Scholar]

Davis, N. (2019). https://www.dataforprogress.org/blog/2019/1/29/unpacking-millennials-racial-attitudes Accessed on 6th May 2022.

DeSante, C & Smith, C. (2020). Racial Stasis: The Millennial Generation and the Stagnation of Racial Attitudes in American Politics. Chicago Scholarship Online. Accessed on 6th May 2022.

European Broadcasting Union, (2016). https://www.ebu.ch/news/2016/04/ebu-launches-generation-what-eur Accessed on 12th May 2022.

Hickman, M & Ryan, L. (2020). The "Irish question": marginalizations at the nexus of sociology of migration and ethnic and racial studies in Britain, Ethnic and Racial Studies, 43:16, 96-114, DOI: 10.1080/01419870.2020.1722194

Lloyd, T. (2022). https://hansard.parliament.uk/commons/2022-03-17/debates/B13B98CE-884F-4F04-A321-58140C2EA97C/IrishDiasporaInBritain

Miles, R. (1982). *Racism and Migrant Labour*. London: Routledge Kegan Paul.

Pew Research. (2009). https://www.pewresearch.org/social-trends/2010/02/24/millennials-confident-connected-open-to-change/ Accessed on 5th May 2022.

Ryan, L. (2007). "Who Do You Think You Are? Irish Nurses Encountering Ethnicity and Constructing Identity in Britain." Ethnic and Racial Studies 30 (3): 416–438.

Ryan, L. (2015). 'It's Different Now': A Narrative Analysis of Recent Irish Migrants Making Sense of Migration and Comparing Themselves with Previous Waves of Migrants." *Irish Journal of Sociology* 23 (2): 114–132.

Ryan, L, and Kurdi, E. (2015). "Always up for the Craic': Young Irish Professional Migrants Narrating Ambiguous Positioning in Contemporary Britain." *Social Identities* 21 (3): 257–272.

Inclusion and Hope:
'Rainbow of the Mind'

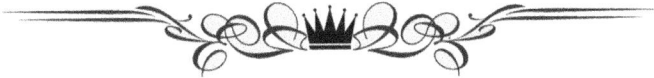

Dr. Phil Noone

"A rainbow is a prism that sends shards of multicoloured light in various directions. It lifts our spirit and makes us think of what is possible. Hope is the same, a personal Rainbow of the Mind"

(Synder, 2002)

Introduction

We live in a chaotic world, where change and uncertainty are part of everyday life, where the search for 'ontological security' (Giddens 2002) often alludes us, but we struggle on regardless. From polluted landscapes that thicken our oceans, to war in Ukraine, trauma post Covid 19 pandemic, rising cost of living, homelessness, it is perhaps easier to focus on global troubles than on hope. Back (2020) suggests that we live in a time that suffers not from doubt but from certainty. In the 1950s, Albert Camus wrote in the conclusion to his essay *The Myth of Sisyphus*, that "hope is a false dichotomy created to help humans cope with the absurdity of existence, we must strive to live rich and meaningful lives, realising that we serve no greater purpose but to live, here and now" (Camus 1955:64,65).

Others have a different view. Sir David Attenborough delivers a message of hope to COP26 Leaders on Climate Change, where he argues, "if we restore the wild, it will help us capture carbon and bring back balance to our planet and thus we must continually work to create a more sustainable, better world" (United Nations Climate Change Conference 2021). Hope is frequently conceptualised as a *future* orientated concept (Snyder 2002), yet, for Back (2020) the role of phenomenology, or lived experience is vital as hope needs to zoom into conditions of the present.

Like seaweed, scattered, tangled along seascapes of the Wild Atlantic Way on the West Coast of Ireland, hope and inclusion, in my opinion, exist in a shifting space of 'temporal tangling'! Developing a hopeful understanding does not deny trouble (Philo & Parr 2019). It concerns not only what is, but also what might be. I argue that hope springs from a rippling attentiveness to our world, to nature, our seascapes, to what exists in the moment. Using narrative data from autoethnography of sea-swimming at Blackrock Diving Tower in Galway, I offer some personal insights into this world of hope, that is collective, connected, inclusive and hopeful in the energy and excitement of now!

So what is Hope?

Henri Desroche (1979) describes hope as a rope. In his study '*The Sociology of Hope*' he describes hope as like the Fakir's rope. The shaman throws the rope into the air and it remains suspended, upright where he throws it. When the humans grab hold of it and pull themselves up, it takes their strain. From a medical sociological and anthropological perspective, hope is a psychosocial resource that is future orientated but is also utilised in the everyday. Hope is dynamic, relational, individual, context dependant, present and future orientated.

Hope and Millennials

A review of 60 research studies with a university student population of young people, showed that hope is linked to increased academic achievement (Feldman et al 2015), autonomous learning, self-esteem and emotional well-being (Chang et al 2019). Therefore, hope is critical to nourish for students, for millennials as they navigate an increasingly uncertain, complex world.

Millennials are those born between 1981 and 1996 (ages 23-38 in 2019). The Deloitte Global 2022 Gen Z and Millennial Survey tells us that Millennials are struggling with financial anxiety while trying to invest in environmentally sustainable choices (https://www2.deloitte.com). We often speak of Millennials as if they were a separate group of people, different to ourselves as older adults. Maybe yes, they are more digital savvy, yet, at the core of every human being is the need to be accepted, to be loved, to feel included, to be part of something! Instead of concentrating in our differences, why not embrace our sameness?

December 12th 2021

I watch in awe. Tall, young, fit, he climbs to the top of the tower. It's cold. Winter. December. I watch as he dives. Somersaults, back flips. Perfection. He joins his friends. They laugh, cheer one another. They all dive. Then swim (PN:480).

At Blackrock Diving Tower in Galway, Ireland, there is a seamless inclusivity of sea swimmers. Shared interest. Common passion. To swim, dive, and feel alive. An article in The Irish Times newspaper (Kelleher 2019) describes the addictive magic of swimming in the sea in winter. As Auerbach de Freitas states "when you're in the water, you stop thinking about anything that might worry you". Cormac Staunton, in this same article, speaks of the "mini-tribes" of people who come to Salthill throughout the year. "You've got the early morning warriors, the people that would be in there at six of clock in the morning, and then you've got the ones who come at five or six in the evening after work. You have the 11.30 crew, which is all the retired guys and older women. To listen to them is a tonic. Sometimes you're walking down there and you hear them laughing and roaring. They're all having the craic. It's life affirming really."

For me, it's this culture of community that makes this place inclusive, special, hopeful.

January 9th 2022

Our Swim Pod 3, formed in 2020, to help us cope with the restrictions and uncertainty of Covid 19 (Phil, NMc and Cliona). Our own sub-cultural group, belonging to the larger cultural group of sea swimmers in Galway.

"We swim. Sea calm. Glistening light of wintery sun dancing on the water as our arms slice through the water with each stroke. Emerging from the water. Cold. We change. Chat. Distracted by a group of 6-8 nearby swimmers. Cheering. Opening a box of chocolates to share with their friends. A Happy Birthday moment. A celebration. During Covid 19. I watch. Silent. The banter and friendliness extending beyond this small group of friends to us and others nearby. The rippling impact of happiness. Of inclusivity. Of catching the moment. I smile. Happy. We chat amongst ourselves. Being 'part of' and yet 'apart from' this moment. This shifting nature of inclusivity. It tangles itself around me. In this space of now. Its simplicity touches me. Their infectious laugher drifts our way. We laugh too. Sharing. A simple moment. Joyful." (PN:560).

What makes this space *special* is this sense 'of knowing and not knowing'. Blackrock Diving Tower is a public space where conversation flows freely, a space where people come to swim and dive and enjoy the seascape in all its guises. A space boundless in its joy, fun and laughter. No questions asked, no dress code. Not everyone uses a 'dry robe'! It doesn't matter. Anything goes. I love the sense of 'non-pretence' that this space offers. People can be just who they are. Pre-swim, we change, heading in. Post-swim, we wrap up warm, share some banter and head home.

March 4th 2021

There is a lightness to the conversational exchange, and, for me, this is special.

"What's the temperature today?" asks NMc, as he spots Paddy emerging from the water. *"7.2 today"*, Paddy replies. *"Are you heading in?"* "We are!" says NMc, as we reluctantly change in the windy gale swirling around us! *We jump into the ocean-black (as it looks today). It's Baltic....! I gasp for breath as the initial cold hits my body and my mind! Momentarily speechless! Numbing of hands. Numbing of feet. Cold extending to my upper chest. Noticing my breath. Fast, short! And then, the sense of settling. Of calmness. As we begin to swim. Checking to make sure we are all OK.* (PN:182).

Just simple fun. Laughter. Encouragement. Looking out for one another. Sharing a similar experience in our own unique way.

January 12ᵗʰ 2022

"Oh, that was great. I'm starving!" she said. "I could eat three dinners", she said. We agreed. 'Sea hunger', we said, as we excitedly hurried into the cold dark waters of the winter's night. (PN: 600)

I recall another day, at lunchtime. It was blustery, cold. The lady who was changing beside me began to chat: "Be sure to put all your clothes securely in your bag when you go in," she said. "When I came out of the water yesterday, my leggings had taken off with the wind, into the sea! I'd to walk to the car with a towel around me. Aye, expensive pair too! It's windy. Aye… your clothes will be gone!" (PN:640)

The normality of this exchange, the sense of looking out for one another, of protecting one another. Just a common shared humanity. And a beautiful one at that!

February 12ᵗʰ 2022

"My identity here feels free, boundless, limitless. No expectation. My time guided by the tides, the look and feel of the ocean. How I feel. My mood. My energy. Knowing that post swim I'll feel elated, calm, energetic, hungry, happy. I sit a moment before I go in. It's sunny. Kinda warm! I think of how Giddens refers to our post-modern existence as living in 'a runaway world'. He's right you know! We're always running and rushing, doing this and that! But here time stops. It's like as if the thoughts in my head are crashing against the walls of my mind, competing with one another, overlapping with one another. Swimming gives them a chance. To slow in the water. To become non-existent. All that exists in the water is the ocean, the sea-weed, the sky blue with its dancing clouds, the sound of rippling, gentle back and forth, the wider seascape, the horizon beyond, the cry of a gull as it darts towards the water to catch a fish. The occasional sound of wild ducks flying overhead. I'm happy sitting here. Reflecting. Writing. Knowing the delight that awaits as I jump into the luminous ocean of today. (PN 780)

November 10th 2021

It's late. Dark. Cliona and I were swimming. We notice a red/yellow shimmer on the water. Mesmerising. A coat of colour. We swam in it, and marvel at its beauty, magnificence. We are awe struck. I just assume it is the reflection of the moon that is catching the street light and reflecting it in this strange and unique way in the water. We are transfixed, moved, excited. To experience this sense of now.

Eventually, we exit the water. Change and as we head up the slight slope at Blackrock, I glance back at the water. The magnificent display of shimmering colour is gone. I comment "Oh it must be the unusual reflection of the light". Think no more about it and head home

Next night, same time. As we change into our swimming gear a Millennial begins conversing with Cliona, who is also a Millennial. Excited. Animated. In full flow. He had just come out of the water. He said "were you in yet?" Cliona: "Not yet. Just heading in." "Did you see it!" he exclaimed. And then he began to explain why the water was a sea of magnificent orange, greens and blues. Bio-luminous algae. My excitement sored. Oh, let me jump in and experience this wonder!

We swam out and there it was! A spectacle of silver dots. Different to the night before. But tantalisingly beautiful. As we dipped our hand into the water, hundreds of silver dots appeared and disappeared. Like the magic of glow worms experienced some years previously in caves in New Zealand. I was astonished. Excited. Afraid to speak. Almost afraid to breathe in case my breath disturbed this wonderous sight. We stayed for ages in the water. Transfixed. Giggling like excited children on bonfire night.

The next night we swam again. Our hearts hopeful we would capture this amazing phenomenon. The sea was a shimmering shade of blue. Bright and dark. Moving, wavering, disappearing, reappearing. We treaded water. Immersed in its colour. Speechless. Lucky. Alive (PN 320).

This intergenerational swimming space, made up of conversation, solitude, silence, togetherness and aloneness. It defies loneliness as it embraces a sharing. It exists as a paradox of spaces. If I chose to exclude myself, am quiet, in need of silence, I find it here. And if I choose to say 'hello' engage in conversation, it is that too and more. The cold Atlantic waters welcomes me, embraces me, holds me, comforts me, surrounds me, entangles me in its waves when its rough and windy, allows me to float in non-existent wonder on serene-sea days. This deep immersive connectedness. Thus, its inclusivity exists as a 'mind-heart-body' connectedness, a deepening of my connectedness to myself, and yet, an expansion of my connectedness to the wider seascape, the sky, the sea weed, the whiteness of the wave tips, the glimmering reflection of the sun catching the water. This experience is different each time I swim. And thus, I love it each time for what it is. Just as it is. In its present-ness. This awareness, to me, is the inclusiveness of the ocean space, which I call 'Ocean Mindfulness'.

This sense of inclusivity, in my opinion, offers hope. Our Swim Pod

3, our banter, craic, fun and engagement. I hear Millennials laugh and joke and I love it. Did you watch the match... and on it goes! All ages swim here. There are no divisions in this space. It's a space for everyone, even the occasional dog comes to swim and say hello!

Conclusion

Using autoethnography allowed me to explore inclusiveness and hope by zooming into a personal embodied experience and zooming out to the wider cultural community of sea swimming. Blackrock Diving Tower is a swimming space shared by all and this includes our beautiful, robust and resilient Millennials. Our youth are the future! Let us honour their strength, their abilities and shift the narrative from one of negativity to create a more inclusive positive space. Long live our Swim Pod 3, with its diversity of age and gender, including our golden, vibrant, positive, resilient Millennial, Cliona, whose laugh rings out to bring a smile and joy to all who are fortunate enough to share in its joy. Let us bring the 'Rainbow of the Mind' into the seascape and enjoy! Let us step gingerly into the ocean or take a dive into the waters below to strengthen our emotional resilience and create a 'pause' from what Giddens so eloquently describes as our uncertain, runaway world. I joke you not, try it, it works!

*If you are new to cold water swimming, be cautious, never swim alone, start in the summer when water temperatures are warmer, swim where a lifeguard is present, check the tides and weather conditions beforehand. Join a more experienced group of sea swimmers. Take care. Always. In water. And enjoy.

References

Attenborough D. (2021) *United Nations Climate Change Conference*. Address to COP26 on Climate Change: Glascow. Available at: http://www.rev.com.transcripts Accessed on 26/04/2022.

Back L. (2020) Hope's work. *Antipode*. 53(1), 3-30.

Camus A. & O Brien J. (1955) *The Myth of Sisyphus and Other Essays*. New York: Knoph.

Chang E. C. & Chang O. D. & Mingqi L. & Shen X. & Yuwei L. & Zhang X. & Wang X. (2019) Positive emotions, hope, and life satisfaction in Chinese adults: A test of the broaden and build model in accounting for subjective well-being in Chinese college students. *The Journal of Positive Psychology*. 14(6), 829-835.

Deloitte Global Gen Z and Millennials Survey (2022) Available at: http://www2.deloitte.com Accessed on 28/06/2022.

Desroche H. (1979) *The Sociology of Hope*. Law Book: Co. of Australasia.

Feldman D. B. & Kubota M. (2015) Hope, self-efficacy, optimism and academic achievement: Distinguishing constructs and levels of specificity in predicting college grade-point average. *Learning and Individual Differences*. 37, 210-216.

Giddens A. (2002) Runaway World. How Globalisation is Reshaping our Lives. London:Profile Books.

Kelleher (2019) The addictive magic of swimming in the sea in winter: 'It's life affirming' *The Irish Times*. Nov 23rd 2019. Available at: http://www.irishtimes.com.

Philo C. & Parr H. (2019) Staying with the trouble of institutions. *Area*. 51(2), 241-249.

Snyder C. R. (2002) Hope theory: Rainbows in the mind. *Psychological Inquiry*. 13(4), 249-275.

Creativity in Social Care:
Promoting A Landscape of Inclusion and Hope

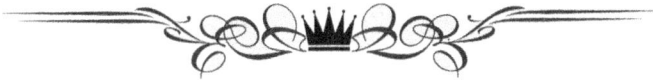

Susan McKenna

Introduction

This chapter looks at the role creativity plays in social care and, more generally, mental health services. It has its basis in training I completed some two decades ago in social care influenced by theorists such as Rogers (1954), Axline (1969) and Winnicott (1971) and, later, systemic family therapy. This is where I became deeply interested in creative ways of working with children, adolescents and their wider families deemed by various authorities to be 'at risk'. Fundamentally, I witnessed how important creative approaches such as art and music were to clients and their families - many who could not articulate how they felt about various past and contemporary traumas in their lives. This is a recurring theme in the literature (Plucker et al., 2004; Rogers, 1954).

Freud originally wrote about trauma in the context of war neurosis, understanding trauma to be a break of the stimulus barrier that overwhelmed the ego. Contemporaneously, social care, as employed with traumatised children and adolescents, seeks to build ego functionality, enhance reality testing, and build frustration tolerance capacity so it has moved on from the original thinking, seeking to include clients in the process of engagement to provide them with hope.

Van der Kolk (1987) suggests that it is when the child or adolescent can bring up and discuss experienced trauma but also, crucially, be capable of conceiving and imagining a range of other things that three things may occur; resolution, neutralisation and synthesis. Trauma should not be underestimated. I experienced this first hand when working with children and adolescents and their teams in several cities in Ireland, Sweden and Canada. Trauma is pervasive in the mind, body and soul of clients who have experienced single and multiple traumas (Levine, 2008; 2010). There is now an established body of evidence confirming traumatic experiences being linked to complex, deep-rooted, emotional and psychological fear resulting in an inability to trust, resulting in a range of attachment issues and anxiety.

Concepts and Constructs of Creativity in Achieving a Landscape of Inclusion and Hope

What exactly is creativity? Schmid (2005: 6) in Val Huet (2012) outlines creativity as, "the innate capacity to think and act in original ways (to the individual person), to be inventive, to be imaginative, and to find new and original solutions to need and forms of expression." Essentially, we attempt to develop and encourage new solutions to old problems. Within this context, co-creation only occurs over a period of time whereby both a safe environment is created for clients and trust is established.

The central difficulty with using the term creativity is that it remains an abstract concept. Thus, creativity is considered a dynamic construct within therapeutic exchanges, but there is a lack of clarity concerning its specific task in child and adolescent counselling (Rouse, Armstrong, & McLeod, 2015). This has resulted in problematic definitional issues in the literature, as expressed by Plucker et al. (2004) where the terms become too fluid for anything definite.

Creativity has been described as 'one of psychology's orphans' due to its relative neglect within counselling research when one compares it to other more dominant themes. There is widespread acknowledgement that creativity in the approach is a positive modality in enhancing the therapeutic relationship (Rogers, 1954). This applies to both the counsellor and the client (Duffey et al., 2009). Runco and Jaeger (2012) engaged a meta-analysis review of the literature in psychology and psychotherapy, looking at commonly used definitions of creativity and reported a consensus that creativity is three things; novel, functional, or adaptive.

'Creative approaches to social care', at the time of my diploma and degree studies, was formally on the social care curricula around the country within the Institutes of Technology. However, it seems fair to argue that it was not taken too seriously by the more academically minded students and, indeed, lecturing staff. It was only after a period of time that the subject was allocated the same number of hours as other more 'relevant' subjects, such as psychology and law. Two decades + experience in direct practice and several supervisory/management positions, have convinced me that when the goals of the client and social care practitioner are in alignment, creativity may flow and amazing results are possible.

Creativity is Borne from Intuition

I subscribe to the view that creativity is borne from intuition and this is something Heidi Messenger, one of the Book Hub authors and I, spent many hours discussing. Thus, it is key the social care practitioner accesses their inner worlds to facilitate an insightful perspective towards engagement and intervention and does not rely solely on often outdated theories that simply do not work in practice. The social care practitioner must remain hopeful of potential change and be inclusive in approach. In this process, the clients must be encouraged to look to their own creative intuition. Possibilities are endless if we believe this to be so.

Why is Creativity Useful in Social Care Practice

I'm consistently surprised that research has only relatively recently sought to identify and confirm the potential benefits of creativity with academic rigor. There is no doubt but that creativity assists in the enhancement of coping skills, in building and maintaining relationships and in ensuring a reciprocal relationship. So, I believe it's not too radical to suggest that creativity resides within every single one of us and, further, that it is a source of hope. The clients we typically work with in social care all too often, come to us as a last port of call when other avenues have been either blocked to them or haven't worked for them (Flaskas et al., 2007). Thus, they require new approaches and new solutions to existing often deep-rooted problems. If they are 'frozen' in their thinking and behaviour talk therapy approaches can appear overly rigid and an effective social care practitioner can use a range of creative approaches such as guided or free play, drama, art or music to name but a few of the tools at their disposal.

In summary, social care practice is a mutually collaborative process inherently creative by nature – if we allow it to be so (Siegel, 2007). Core to leveraging creativity exists with the social care practitioner founded on a desire to access their own personal sources of creativity. Creativity may be understood as a conscious act of combining inspiration and insight based on a theoretical understanding of the efficacy of different approaches to client work. A practical example of this is with a young client with whom I worked. He was extremely difficult to engage, on any level, but I noticed he was crazy about Elvis Presley, always listening to his music whenever there was a lull in formal activity programmes. We decided to paint a poster of Elvis and, after some reluctance, he participated, found he loved it and this wonderfully facilitated his artistic expression. We all have it in us…

Concluding Comments

The literature and my experience training and lecturing on various programmes over the years, confirm that creativity is a composite part of human consciousness and behaviour. If a social care practitioner can use creative approaches in our client work, it increases the capacity for moment-by-moment functioning. By this I mean, being 'in' the moment with a client. A safe and secure therapeutic space allows for the active exploration of feelings and emotions which may be too difficult to articulate. Social care is a way of working that allows mistakes and readjustments in approach so that current ways of thinking and behaving can be explored, addressed, and challenged to achieve new ways of thinking and doing. It is by its very nature a co-creative relationship and experience.

Indeed, I came across a lovely quote from van der Kolk (2014: 275), who observes:

> *"Most traditional therapies downplay or ignore the moment-to-moment shifts in our inner sensory world."*

*The author acknowledges the pioneering work of John Hanna and the Limerick City Youth Encounter Project where she first formally experienced the value of creativity and hope for children and adolescents and their families.

References

Axline, V. M. (1947). Play therapy. New York, NY: Ballantine Books.

Axline, V. M. (1969). Play therapy (Rev. ed.). New York, NY: Ballantine Books.

Carson, D., & Becker, K. (2004). When lightning strikes: Reexamining creativity in psychotherapy. *Journal of Counseling & Development, 82*(1), 111-115. doi: 10.1002/j.1556-6678.2004.tb00292.x

Duffey, T., Haberstroh, S., & Trepal, H. (2009). A grounded theory of relational competencies and creativity in counseling: Beginning the dialogue. *Journal of Creativity in Mental Health, 4*(2), 89-112.doi: 10.1080/15401380902951911.

Flaskas, C. (2007). Holding hope and hopelessness: Therapeutic engagements with the balance of hope. Journal of Family Therapy. 29. 186 - 202. 10.1111/j.1467-6427.2007.00381.x.

Levine, K. & Levine, E. (Eds.). (2004). Foundations of expressive arts therapy: Theoretical and clinical perspectives. London: Jessica Kingsley Publishers.

Levine, E. (2003). Tending the fire. Studies in art, therapy and creativity. London: EGS Press.

Levine, P. (2008). Healing trauma: A pioneering program for restoring the wisdom of your body. Boulder, Colorado: Sounds True, Inc.

Levine, P. (2010). In an unspoken voice: How the body releases trauma and restores goodness. Berkeley, California: North Atlantic Books.

Levine, S. (2018). Polyvagal Theory and trauma. In S. W. Porges & D. Dana (Eds.), *Clinical applications of the polyvagal theory* (3-26). New York, NY: W.W. Norton & Company.

Plucker, J. A., Beghetto, R. A., & Dow, G. T. (2004). Why isn't creativity more important to educational psychologists? Potentials, pitfalls, and future directions in creativity research. *Educational Psychologist, 39*(2), 83-96.

Porges, S. W., Doussard-Roosevelt, J. A., & Maiti, A. K. (1994). Vagal tone and the physiological regulation of emotion. *Monographs of the Society for Research in Child Development,* 59(2-3), 250-283. https://dx.doi.org/10.2307/1166144

Rogers, C. R. (1954). Toward a theory of creativity. *Etc: A Review of General Semantics, 11*(4), 249–260.

Rouse, A., Armstrong, J., & McLeod, J. (2015). Enabling connections: Counsellor creativity and therapeutic practice. *Counselling and Psychotherapy Research, 15*(3), 171-179.doi: 10.1002/capr.12019

Runco, M. A., & Jaeger, G. J. (2012). The standard definition of creativity. *Creativity Research Journal, 24*(1), 92–96. https://doi.org/10.1080/10400419.2012.650092

Schaefer, C.E. (2003). Foundations of play therapy. Hoboken, New York: J. Wiley.

Schmid T, ed (2005) Promoting health through creativity for professionals in healthcare arts and education. London: Whurr.

Schmid T, ed (2005) Promoting health through creativity for professionals in healthcare arts and education. London: Whurr.

Siegel, D.J. (1999). The developing mind: How relationships and the brain interact to shape *who we are*. New York: Guilford Press. Smith, J.A., Flowers, P., & Larkin, M. (2009).

Siegel, D. J. (2007). The mindful brain: Reflection and attunement in the cultivation of well- being. New York, New York: W. W. Norton & Company, Inc.

Siegel, D.J. & Bryson, T.P. (2012). The Whole-Brain Child: 12 Proven Strategies to Nurture your Child's Developing Mind. London: Robinson.

Siegel, D. & Solomon, M. (Eds.). (2003). *Healing trauma and attachment, mind, body, and brain*. New York, New York: W. W. Norton & Company.

van der Kolk, R. A. (1987). Psychological trauma. Washington, DC: American Psychiatric Press.

van der Kolk, B. (2005). Developmental trauma disorder: Toward a rational diagnosis for children with complex trauma histories. *Psychiatric Annals, 35,* 401- 405.

van der Kolk, B. A. (2014). The body keeps the score: Brain, mind, and body in the healing of trauma. New York, New York: Viking.

Val Huet (2012). Creativity in a cold climate: Art therapy-based organisational consultancy within public healthcare, International Journal of Art Therapy, 17:1,25-33, DOI: 10.1080/17454832.2011.653649

Winnicott, D. W. (1971). Playing and reality. New York: Basic Books.

The Soul's Journey is as Unique as the Individual Soul

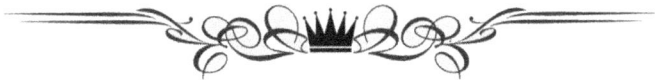

Dr. Mary Helen Hensley

Introduction

It is with such a mixed bag of really cool emotions that I write this piece on hope and inclusion. I chose today, the first day of Pride month June 2022, to sit down and attempt to wax lyrical on a topic that is near and dear to my heart. As the Head of Diversity, Inclusion and Equality for the small, yet powerfully vociferous indie publishing house that is Book Hub Publishing, I am always searching for new ways to address age old conflicts with fresh and thought-provoking perspectives. To be honest, I cringed a little when the theme I was given included 'hope'. Like so many words which have been situationally hammered into mere shadows of their original meaning, I would tend to side with the prolific words of actor, Jim Carrey, when he addressed the graduating class of MIU in 2014.

"I don't believe in hope. Hope is a beggar. Hope walks through the fire and faith leaps over it. You can spend your whole life imagining ghosts and worrying about the pathway to the future, but all there will ever be is what's happening here and the decisions we make this moment. Magic happens when you stop hoping and start knowing."

Help Other People Evolve

I have also heard hope described as H.O.P.E. - *Help Other People Evolve.* On first glance, it sounds good, like a nice phrase one might see on social media, super-imposed over a picture of a pretty rainbow, or birds flying in perfect formation, or two hands, expectantly clasped in unity. I can't say I really like what that implies, however, because right or wrong, I think evolution of the mind, the heart and the process of awakening consciousness, is an incredibly personal journey. The unfurling of an individual's understanding of diversity, inclusion and equality, is often a necessarily painful progression, both in the giving and receiving.

Recently, I had a terribly curious conversation with someone who had lost a significant amount of weight in the past few years. Laughing at the ridiculous nature of her own words, she explained that after working hard to achieve her 'ideal' body size, she found herself exasperated, *grossed-out* even, by 'fat' people. The 'help other people evolve' concept of providing hope to others who often ask how she lost the weight, by her own confession, irritates her. The expectation that all humans equally possess the same band-width, or desire to help others, is, in itself, a lofty aspiration. I pointed out, what seemed to me, to be the obvious. She had literally become the proverbial shoe on the other foot. I asked if it had occurred to her that others, who considered themselves more fit, more vigilant with their diets, more diligent with body movement, when *she* had been obese, might possibly have held the exact same feelings towards her that she now held towards those who were *larger* than her? Again, she laughed, and assured me that she was *certain* this was the case. She regaled me with tales of when she had been teased, fat shamed, and had a very poor sense of self-esteem, due to her size. One might automatically assume that this experience, followed by her recent weight-loss and boosted sense of positive body image, would naturally place her in the evolutionary position of *cheerleader* or *motivator* to those who wished to follow a similar path. It's interesting how we make those assumptions. It was in this revelation, that the 'hope is a beggar' statement really hit home for me.

To assume that everyone who was picked last for the team, has been on the receiving end of harsh judgements, bad behaviour, careless whispers or bullying, will eventually mature and evolve into someone who is principled, supportive and all-inclusive is an act of folly, in my opinion. It creates an 'outside-in' expectation that happiness, self-security and feelings of belonging are things that rely on the tools and skills, (or lack-there-of), of a confused, hurt, fickle and unpredictable population of fledgling, post-modern human beings.

Eight billion plus humans are currently working on eight billion plus storylines, some similar, many very different, all with a variety of characters and situations; personal, generational, cultural, political, socio-economic, stress-causing and privilege varied. To hope, assume even, that the inevitable lessons of life will automatically cause one to take up a cause, donning the 'breastplate of righteousness', makes about as much sense as expecting a young child who has managed to add 2+2, to instinctively move on to more advanced calculations. For some, 2+2 is as much as they can manage within their inimitable circumstances.

Dr. Mary Helen Hensley

The Soul's Journey is as Unique as the Individual Soul

In thirty years of work in metaphysics, and twenty-five as a Doctor of Chiropractic, I have come to realise that the soul's journey is as unique as the individual soul, itself. Every single inhabitant of this beautiful planet of ours, is here to experience, work through, implement or discard, a multitude of interactions, physical, emotional and spiritual, inside a variety of perfectly orchestrated boxes. As we grow through some pleasurable and often horrible interactions during our time here on earth, I think we have become a bit careless with our expectations that everyone can or *should* grow at the same rate. There are some, in my years of experience of intimate, one on one work with my fellow travellers, who take a lifetime, to execute a single, or a series of lessons that may result in their understanding of what it means to be human. There are others, who are able to release trauma, anger, guilt or shame at a much more rapid pace. These individuals are far more likely to imbibe a sense of moral obligation to champion ideals such as the celebration of diversity, or to strive to always be inclusive.

Jim Carrey told his captive audience of promising new graduates that "magic happens when you stop hoping and start knowing." I genuinely believe that this is one of the soundest pieces of advice I've ever heard. To *know* the world in which we live, to embrace the understanding that inclusion is not a given in any life scenario…this is where the magic begins. When people crave inclusion, it means that some part of them has yet to understand that acceptance, validation, confirmation and support must first come from within. To adhere to the trauma of being on the outside, of not fitting in, of not being treated equally as one perceives others to be treated, can be a slippery slope. Imagine, instead, the brave soul who recognises that every last morsal of

32

experience in this world is based on the synergistic exchange of frequency and the energy we personally project into any given situation.

Imagine the soul who dares to love itself, to honour its own unique journey; the one who encourages itself to risk hurt, isolation and heartbreak in exchange for the possibility, the opportunity to love and be loved by others. By the iron-clad universal laws of energetic and spiritual dynamics, said soul will begin to attract other people and experiences that are in alignment *with the work they are willing to put in,* to make manifest their desires for inclusion and equality.

Sometimes this happens slowly, but surely, and other times, it happens at lightning speed, and voilà…hope becomes knowing, like an alchemist turns lead into gold.

My personality is such that I tend to always expect an amazing outcome to every challenge. My life to date, however, has re-defined my definition of amazing. The least painful, easiest outcomes are sometimes the solution, but I have found that more so than not, the meat and potatoes are found within the difficult and awkward. I was adjusting spines, healing with frequency, writing books about returning from death, and raising the children I had out of wedlock, by myself, in a foreign country. I know a little bit about exclusion. My livelihood was threatened by throwaway statements from medical professionals who knew nothing of my qualifications as a doctor.

When I first began to realise that I had a child who was moving towards bi-sexuality, I was the one who became uncomfortable when we would read bedtime stories that inevitably ended with the happily ever after of a prince and princess. Rather than gripe about the non-inclusive nature of the old-school fairy tales, I began writing a series of books in which *every* child could see themselves. It was only those uncomfortable feelings of exclusion that prompted me to create something new.

The idea of wishing or hoping for a perfect world in which everyone can simply be who they are, is to exclude the pivotal moments that are responsible for creating the momentum behind the changes we wish to see. Inclusion begins in the heart, then spreads into the everyday mannerisms and deeds of the individual, which in turn begins to generate its own powerful field of attraction, which opens up channels of grace and opportunity, that would otherwise be unattainable.

Feeding Hope: Millennials and Food Sustainability

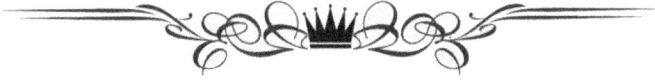

Cathy Fitzgibbon aka "The Culinary Celt"

"The tiny seed knew that in order to grow, it needed to be dropped in dirt, covered in darkness and struggle to reach the light"
— Sandra King.

Holding onto Hope

Science and experience tell us that seeds will grow, but it's also fair to add that, when initially planted in the soil the hope of a plentiful harvest is also always sown. In recent years, many different parts of the world and its emerging Millennial generation population, have been hit by a multitude of major distresses ranging from political conflicts, unsettling weather patterns, droughts and rising sea levels, to food and fuel price increases. If not addressed, this type of man-made destruction will further very significantly escalate food in-equality gaps. In this regard, Shenggen *et al.,* (2014) maintain that the magnitude of these types of global issues, during turbulent times, will leave disadvantaged communities increasingly vulnerable to the threat of emerging diseases and contaminated foods. On a micro-level this will have devastating long-term effects for many households and families in under-developed regions, whilst simultaneously on a macro-level presenting our society as a whole with enormous worldwide food shortages. To this effect Millennials have much to say and contribute. In fact, the Deloitte Global Millennial Survey (2021) suggests that the pandemic, extreme climate events, and a charged socio-political atmosphere may in actual fact have reinforced their passions and given them oxygen.

The Food and Agriculture Organization (1996) links the existence of food security to physical and economic access to adequate amounts of nutritious, safe and culturally appropriate food to maintain a healthy and active life. More recently, Fahy (2021) concurs that food security is the measure of an individual's ability to access food that is both nutritious and sufficient in quantity. According to the Global Food Security Index (2021), Ireland is ranked the most food secure country in the world scoring highly on all four pillars of food security: affordability, availability, quality and safety, natural resources and resilience. However, Tutty (2022) draws attention to the fact that, like much of the rest of the word, Ireland's food security is now also under pressure due to knock-on effects of the war in Ukraine and increasingly fragile global supply chain logistics. Glauber and Laborde (2022), for example, acknowledge the recent conflict between Russia and the Ukraine as having a huge impact on global food supply chains with the exports of these two countries, referred to as the 'Europe's breadbasket', representing 12% of all food calories traded in the world. Likewise for hundreds of millions of people in other countries such as Somalia and Yemen this right is continually not being met due to a combined mixture of external factors outside of their control, such as availability and access to food, stability from climate change and political instability (Concern, 2021).

The Food and Agriculture Organization of the United Nations (2021) acknowledges that we are at a critical juncture in terms of the number of people in the world affected by hunger, having increased in 2020 under the shadow of the COVID-19 pandemic. Their acknowledgement highlights figures of between 720 and 811 million people being faced with hunger, after remaining virtually unchanged from 2014 to 2019. However, on a more positive note, amidst this backdrop worldwide uncertainty, food also has the intrinsic ability to bring both comfort and hope to the emerging Millennial cohort. Fitzgibbon and MacGiolla Bhuí (2019) reveal that Millennials are increasingly shaping their food conversations online by asking core questions about their food sources and it's these important long-term questions that will ultimately sustain their overall sense of health and happiness into the future. Thus, reaffirming the power that the physical ability of food strives to bring hope into the future, alongside the day-to-day joy in keeping us healthy and alive.

Planting Hope

The vocation of farming truly **epitomises** the pursuit of hope. Hayden (2021) concurs that without hope and persistence, it would not be possible for these men and women to continue to work or enter this profession. Having grown up on a farm it's been fascinating to experience first-hand the seasonal planting of seeds, with hope of a fruitful harvest, by both my grandparents and parents. This combination of both their love of nature and the ingrained sense of hope makes it easy for me to relate to the fact that holding onto and maintaining it in this occupation can at times be extremely exciting, whilst at the same time equally challenging. However, as crops begin to grow and prosper from season to season so, too, does confidence. Families from generation-to-generation and entire communities can thrive in the knowledge that the future they hope for is safe and secure.

Fortunately, in this fast-paced digital-first era, Millennials are also increasingly passionate about farming and are extremely keen to know how and where their food is produced. The concept of sustainable farming is thankfully embedded in the DNA of this 'foodie' generation bringing with it a sense of optimism and hope in the form of believing that they have the power to effect change. Mesesan supports the view that Millennials are actively leading the movement toward a more *organic agricultural* system, with over 50% of this cohort in the U.S. actively incorporating organic foods in their diet (www.greenmoney.com).

With the age range of Millennials now being 19-39 this cohort can no longer be labelled a 'young generation'. Being one of the largest generational cohorts they are now reaching their prime working and spending years, with the oldest almost turning 40! Being fully immersed in the workforce they've taken up the mantle in the agricultural sector in terms of revolutionising the future of farming (Walch, 2019). In this respect, positive figures from the Census of Agriculture (2020) show a slight increase in the proportion of farm holders in Ireland under the age category of 35 between 2010 and 2020. The use of modern and emerging agricultural and AI technologies can help bring about positive shifts in how they view farming today. Havyas (2020) indicates that attracting these bright minds into this profession will be of paramount importance to help solve the problems of world food insecurity and global hunger by moving from traditional ways to more modern farming methods, that will make agriculture even more efficient and sustainable, a point also noted by Hayden (2022) in this book.

In recent times sustainability can very much be thrown around as a buzz word! According to Dowling (2020), it's important to note that sustainability focuses on meeting the needs of the present while also ensuring the ability of future generations to meet their needs encompassing three key elements: economy, environment and society. Wilde (2021) suggests that as food provides a link between the population health, food security and environmental sustainability agendas it is of paramount importance that this highly influential cohort maintains an all-encompassing perspective of the role it plays in understanding the true meaning of sustainability, and actioning on it to radiate hope across all of these fronts when it comes to food.

Harnessing Hope

Millennials are leading the way when it comes to transforming food systems and understanding the complex realities of food production. They are enabling these transformative processes by actively being part of fair, inclusive and equitable systems that promote evenly shared food resources for all. These factors have the ability to influence their buying decisions and shines a light on the way they favour brands committed to fair trade and environmentally sustainable growing practices. Food movements such as Fairtrade have been around for their entire lifespan. Being one of the most recognised and trusted sustainability labels in the world, Fairtrade is co-owned by more than 1.8 million farmers and workers who earn fairer prices, enabling them to build stronger communities which offers them more control over their futures (www.fairtrade.net). Having grown up in an age where ethical buying is not viewed as some type of marketing ploy or add-on, rather an expectation, has enabled the Millennial generation cohort to effectively embrace these types of food movements, ensuring a fairer society when it comes to the food they buy and consume.

Increased awareness of the seasons and the ways in which nature effects our food systems are also key to the sustainability of food sources (Fitzgibbon, 2019). The concept of seasonal eating simply breaks down what we eat each season to maintain health. Then, along with the health benefits seasonal foods are also far better for the environment. On the other hand, foods grown out of season are not able to follow their natural growing and ripening rhythms which can in turn affect their nutritional content. So, eating high-quality seasonal food types with adequate amounts of vitamins, minerals and antioxidants can help nourish, protecting the body and mind from different types of stresses and looks to both physical and mental health. On this front, my debut book 'Eat With The Seasons' showcases the health benefits of various food types according to each season. It is this type of mindful eating education around food that will help empower consumers with practical and meaningful ways to self-reflect and recognise their own personal eating patterns in tune with nature and the four varied seasons of the year, enabling a more overall positive relationship with food (Fitzgibbon, 2022). Thus, the ability for everyone to have access to healthy food sources will depend on the inclusive systems, embraced by all.

Nurturing Hope

Climate change and global warming are unquestionably critical issues that we are all currently faced with, creating with them further challenges for Millennials and upcoming generations to overcome. Due to their life expectancy, Falke *et al.*, (2021) maintain that these later born generations will be much more affected by the climate change compared to their predecessors. The changing climate also makes weather patterns less predictable with some traditional tried and trusted methods of growing crops beginning to fail small-scale farmers and local producers. With this in mind solutions such as sustainable consumption will be one of the ways forward for this generation, to help to support more inclusive, fair and equitable worldwide food structures. Being a large part of the landscape in terms of their buying behaviour influence this generational cohort are no different to the generations that have come before and after them.

However, Falke *et al.,* (2021) deep-dive and further highlight the high importance Millennials place on being in control when purchasing sustainable goods. This extremely heart-warming change is being acknowledged by Millennial consumers, as the market for sustainable products has been steadily growing around the world for more than a decade (Brach *et al.*, 2018).

Furthermore, sustainable consumption simultaneously optimises environmental, social and economic consequences that relate to consumption regarding the needs of current and future generations. So, figuring out a secure, sustainable and fair food system for our planet has become one of the most defining issues of our time and Millennials are taking a lead in this evolution (Fitzgibbon, 2021). Thankfully, in line with this, other additional solutions, such as seasonal eating the above-mentioned sustainable food consumption are currently being addressed by this generation. In my chapter titled "Millennial Culinary Curiosity: Generation Foodie Fuelling Generation Next" in Vol.3 of this book series I touched on the fact that by demanding better food choices from environmentally conscious and ethical sources Millennial consumers are mobilising this cultural movement into their day-to-day activities making food systems more equitable (Fitzgibbon, 2019).

"Every generation must recognize and embrace the task it is peculiarly designed by history and by providence to perform"
— Chinua Achebe.

Some Top Take Aways Tips for Millennials

❖ *Surrender to the Concept of Real Sustainability* – Scratch beneath the surface and better understand and embrace honest and trustworthy ethical food choices. Cut through the marketing of brands and discover what's truly in their DNA.

❖ *Take a Seasonal Eating Approach* - The Celt Mindful Eating Model framework I developed in my book 'Eat With The Seasons' is an easy one to remember: The **C** stands for 'Consider your Food Source', the **E** 'Enjoy and Be Present'; the **L** represents 'Love your Food' and **T** represents how important it is to 'Take notice of your feelings' when it comes to food. This framework in its entirety is designed to help instil a greater sense of daily gratitude and joy drawing from the nurturing ebb and flow of the seasonal cycles.

❖ *Engage all of the Senses* – When it comes to engaging the 5 senses (sight, hearing, smell, touch and taste) in relation to food embracing, the concept of mindful eating can help with the day-to-day figuring out of which foods bring the most pleasure and joy. This, in turn, ultimately creates hope in terms of individual wellbeing, as well as the improved future of our planet as a whole.

❖ *Tune into Technology* - Download and use food waste apps. With so much food going to waste annually these apps help greatly in the reduction in food waste by facilitating the buying and collection of it, at reasonable prices, so it gets eaten rather than wasted.

❖ *Consider Farming as a Career* – We need more guardians of the planet. This profession can be very rewarding on many levels. There are lots of different avenues to consider and lots of supports out there for young budding entrepreneurs.

References

Brach, S., Walsh, G. and Shaw, D. (2018). Sustainable Consumption and Third-party Certification Labels: Consumers' Perceptions and Reactions. *European Management Journal,* 36(2), pp. 254–265. http://eprints.gla.ac.uk/138134/7/138134.pdf

Census of Agriculture. (2020). Preliminary Results. Demographic Profile of Farm Holders. https://www.cso.ie/en/releasesandpublications/ep/p-coa/censusofagriculture2020-preliminaryresults/demographicprofileoffarmholders/

Concern. (2021). These are the world's 10 hungriest countries in 2021. https://www.concernusa.org/story/worlds-hungriest-countries/

Deloitte. (2021). A call for accountability and action. The Deloitte Global 2021 Millennial and Gen Z Survey. https://www2.deloitte.com/content/dam/Deloitte/global/Documents/2021-deloitte-global-millennial-survey-report.pdf

Dowling, C. (2020). Sustainability in Irish Agriculture. *Teagasc.* https://www.teagasc.ie/publications/2020/sustainability-in-irish-agriculture.php

Fahy, A. (2021). What is food security? *Concern Worldwide.* https://www.concern.net/news/what-food-security

Fairtrade. https://www.fairtrade.net/

Falke, A., Schröder, N. and Hofmann, C. (2021). The Influence of Values in Sustainable Consumption Among Millennials. *Journal of Business Economics.* https://link.springer.com/article/10.1007/s11573-021-01072-7.

Fitzgibbon, C. (2022). *Eat With The Seasons.* Galway: Book Hub Publishing.

Fitzgibbon, C. (2021). *Mental Health for Millennials*, (Vol. 5), Galway: Book Hub Publishing.

Fitzgibbon, C. (2019). *Mental Health for Millennials,* (Vol. 3), Galway: Book Hub Publishing.

Fitzgibbon, C. and MacGiolla Bhuí, N. (2019). Millennial Culture, Food and the Pursuit of Happiness. *A #CulinaryCurious Blog.*

https://www.bookhubpublishing.com/2019/06/06/millennial-culture-food-and-the-pursuit-of-happiness/

Food and Agriculture Organization of the United Nations. (2021). The world is at a critical juncture. *The State of Food Security and Nutrition in the World.* https://www.fao.org/state-of-food-security-nutrition

Food and Agriculture Organization. (1996). An Introduction to the Basic Concepts of Food Security. Food Security Information for Action Practical Guides. *EC – FAO Food Security Programme.* al936e00.pdf (fao.org)

Glauber, J. and Laborde, D. (2022). How will Russia's invasion of Ukraine affect global food security? *International Food Policy Research Institute.* https://www.ifpri.org/blog/how-will-russias-invasion-ukraine-affect-global-food-security

Global Food Security Index. (2021). Rankings and trends. Explore the year-on-year trends for the Global Food Security Index. *The Economist Group.* https://impact.economist.com/sustainability/project/food-security-index/Index

Havyas, K S. (2020). Millennials and Gen Z To Revolutionize The Future of Farming. *LinkedIn.* Millennials and Gen Z To Revolutionize The Future of Farming (linkedin.com)

Hayden, A. (2022). *Mental Health for Millennials*, (Vol. 6), Galway: Book Hub Publishing.

Hayden, A. (2021). *Mental Health for Millennials*, (Vol. 5), Galway: Book Hub Publishing.

Mesesan, C. Sustainable Agriculture Outlook Rooted with Millennials. https://greenmoney.com/sustainable-agriculture-outlook-rooted-with-millennials/

Shenggen, F., Rajul, PL., Yosef, S. (2014). Resilience for food and nutrition security. *International Food Policy Research Institute.* http://dx.doi.org/10.2499/9780896296787

Tutty, S. (2022). Ireland facing rationing as Ukraine war hits food and energy supplies. *The Times.* https://www.thetimes.co.uk/article/ireland-facing-rationing-as-ukraine-war-hits-food-and-energy-supplies-hj52jrx6x

Walch, K. (2019). How AI Is Transforming Agriculture. *Forbes.*
https://www.forbes.com/sites/cognitiveworld/2019/07/05/how-ai-is-
transforming-agriculture/#9f7dff84ad10

Wilde, J. (2011). Food Security on the Island of Ireland: Are we Sleepwalking
into a Crisis? *Institute of Public Health in Ireland.*
https://www.publichealth.ie/files/file/Publications/Food%20Security%20on%20t
he%20island%20of%20Ireland%20IPH%20March%202011.pdf

Highway to Hell Health

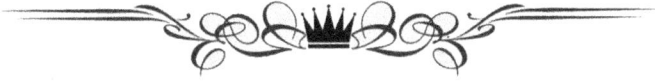

John Madden

One of the greatest changemakers of our time, Desmond Tutu once said that, *"Hope is being able to see that there is light despite all of the darkness"*. It would be difficult to find a more fitting quote when discussing the topic of mental health, or more so, the concept of recovery. At times, a mental illness can be likened to a journey; it has a beginning, middle and ideally, the final destination of wellness. The journey is never a straight line, it can meander so frequently you almost feel as though you are back where you started. You are met with cul-de-sac's, bumpy roads, barriers, diversions, and inadequate or confusing signposting. That's just the route, your vehicle, in essence, the self, will encounter the ups and downs of life too, often culminating in the odd tire or even a breakdown.

However, throughout all of the aforementioned, there is always hope. The Irish mental health services, and many others across the world have adopted the model of recovery to assist people with this journey. Mala et al assert that until the 1970s, many clinicians and mental health professionals believed that persons with mental health conditions were doomed to live with their illness forever and would never really be able to have a fulfilling life which, as you read it, seems beyond hopeless. As with many countries up to then and beyond, one of Ireland's biggest issues in mental health provision, was the over-reliance on the medical model of care which, in itself is, effective to a point. Back to my transport analogies, the medical model focuses on correcting a wrong but doesn't really take the person into consideration, nor does it really get to the root of the issue. It can mask the symptoms and the person can generally lead a meaningful and purposeful life as a result, but to truly treat the person and their issues involves a great deal more work. In essence, the medical model treats the symptoms and the illness, whereas the recovery model treats the person.

According to Jacob (2015), the recovery model is based on two simple premises:

1. It is possible to recover from a mental health condition.
2. The most effective recovery is patient-directed.

The term "patient-directed" is as it sounds, it puts the power and choice back into their hands, very much in-keeping with the Latin idiom, "Nihil de nobis, sine nobis" - nothing about us, without us. It ensures autonomy and independence rather than being told expressly what to do, or even how to live our life. Essentially, it is empowering and puts the person enduring difficulties back in the driving seat. It is always important to remember that, when people find themselves in crisis, that they often feel as though they have little to no meaningful influence over what is going on in their lives. Thus, returning that element of control can be exceptionally beneficial to their individual recovery, almost as though they regain the power to navigate their own lives. It is emancipating and above all else, it works!

The Recovery Model as coined by Leamy et al (2011) is easy to remember as it has five tenets that can be laid out using the word CHIME which, on a personal level, is a reminder of how sound resonates and can be heard by others, The acronym stands for:

- Connectedness
- Hope (And optimism)
- Identity
- Meaning
- Empowerment

Connectedness – Having peer support and social groups, relationships, support from others, and, having a place and purpose in the community. This is something that everybody needs, the opposite of which is of course, isolation. Isolation can be dangerous, especially when trying to traverse a journey to wellness. We are social beings and thrive on meaningful engagement and interaction. When we don't have such basic support, we are prone to excessively unhealthy overthinking, where we often stew in our own juices, or catastrophise the worst possible outcomes to issues. This, in turn, lends itself to further anxieties. Thus, the spiral of misery continues. No one is an island, be they be introverted or extroverted. Although many people do prefer solitude, we all need social outlets to some extent, because being a part of something bigger than ourselves gives our lives purpose.

Hope (and Optimism) – Belief in recovery, motivation to change, hope-inspiring relationships, having dreams and aspirations. What are we without hope? If we have none, there is no motivation and as a result, life seems bleak and pointless. The person enduring the issues may be wholly incapable of seeing any form of hope, and at this point, giving up is the easy solution but to do so, just makes things spiral even further into abject nihilism. That is why the connectedness and other aspects of the model are crucial. Each tenet has a distinct purpose, and like the most intricate of mechanisms, if one part fails, If the person at the centre of this cannot find hope, it can be up to the others involved in the recovery process to try to be the beacon in the darkness, show the way and escort the person to a place of hope, but it needs to be a 50-50 effort with mutual understandings.

Identity - Rebuilding a positive sense of identity and overcoming stigma. Our identity is who we are, and while we have so many commonalities, we are still individuals. Almost like a deck of cards, on the surface, we are a box of 52 cards, but we can be dealt any kind of unique hand. But you might say, 52 cards could hardly have that many combinations...? Would you believe me if I told you there is, wait for it, drum roll please...

80,658,175,170,943,878,571,660,636,856,403,
766,975,289,505,440,883,277,824,000,000,000,000

combinations. So, like the deck of cards, we are all made of the same stuff, but the amalgamation of our individual traits is what sets us all apart. As a result, we have our own unique identity, what makes you, you, and what makes me, me! Those who endure mental health issues nearly all feel as though they are losing who they are as they withdraw from their usual behaviours and outlets, live more insular lives, and can be crippled with anxiety and depression, and more. The self can become unrecognisable and losing that self-identity can take a long time to claw back.

Meaning – Finding meaning in the mental health experience, a meaningful life and social roles, meaningful life and social goals. A life without meaning or purpose is an empty experience, we all need to be a part of something, otherwise, what's the point? When we talk about meaning, it has several connotations; there must be meaning to the journey of recovery so that all involved are cognisant of why we are on this path and where our destination lies. Additionally, the goal is to empower the individual to be able to stand autonomously so that they can reach a point where they can live a life free from the shackles of what has been weighing them down for so long. Eventually, they can get to a stage where they can start planning so that they can further themselves in life, whether that means taking the plunge of trying a new career, course, or even a new routine. Aspirations for a better standard quality of life encapsulate hope. It may take some time to get to this point, after all, much of the work to be done is initially inward but that doesn't mean that we should not encourage aspiration and looking with a more outward perspective. The end-goals may be significant but to help stay the course, break it down into small achievable steps. In doing so, progress can be made at a pace that suits the individual, and every little milestone celebrated and acknowledged. Take for example, the notion of New Years' resolutions, we opt for something and generally it is dropped by mid-January, why you may ask? We were probably setting sights too high. So instead of saying "This year I'm going to run the Dublin City Marathon", don't! Instead, break it down and try saying, by the end of January, I'd like to be able to run for 10 minutes without struggling for breath, maybe February, it could be 20 minutes. That's a lot more achievable than trying to set out to run 26 miles from the get-go!

Empowerment - Personal responsibility, control over life, focusing upon strengths. This is where we want to help the person get to a point where they can stand by themselves. That is not to say that the person is fully recovered or free from the issues that placed them in turmoil in the first instance. Those thoughts can creep back at any stage but through the recovery journey, it is hope that the person now will have garnered greater coping skills; be able to identify those unhelpful thoughts before they become problematic; not be reluctant to seek help when needed; reach out to people rather than languishing alone, becoming overwhelmed by their problems, or even stewing in their own juices.

Recovery is possible and hope is the cornerstone of the process. It is a journey, but rarely a linear one. However, once our vehicle is ready, and we have an idea of the roads to take, the destination is one of the best places to be. It's an interesting journey, on which we can meet some amazing people and learn from them too. Be prepared for heavy traffic at times, and other times, open roads. It will take its toll but you will get there, after all, as Laozi stated, "*A journey of a thousand miles begins with a single step*". Stay going, you'll get there.

References

Jacob KS. Recovery model of mental illness: A complementary approach to psychiatric care. *Indian J Psychol Med.* 2015;37(2):117-119. doi:10.4103/0253-7176.155605

Leamy, M., Bird, V., Le Boutillier, C., Williams, J., and Slade, M. (2011). 'A conceptual framework for personal recovery in mental health: systematic review and narrative synthesis', *British Journal of Psychiatry*, 199(6), pp. 445–452.

Malla A, Joober R, Garcia A. Mental illness is like any other medical illness: A critical examination of the statement and its impact on patient care and society. *J Psychiatry Neurosci.* 2015;40(3):147-150. doi:10.1503/jpn.150099

Sport is not just for the Talented, the Champions and the Early Developers: Creating a Climate of Hope and Inclusion

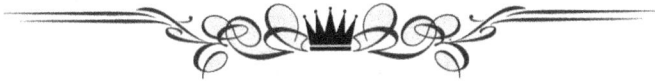

Paul Kilgannon

We are living through a time where the constructs of hope and inclusion are being deeply challenged. The global Covid 19 pandemic has seen many of us lose hope. The ongoing war in the Ukraine is the antithesis of inclusion. The world, and its inhabitants, are experiencing great challenge.

Somewhat ironically, attacks on hope and inclusion highlight and magnify their value; without them...there is suffering.

I am a sports coach and work and write in the area of coach and athlete development. Hope and inclusion are integral in a healthy sporting environment. Hope is what motivates athletes to practice, and what draws them to the competitive environment. Inclusion...that sense of belonging...is what drives courageous effort and performance and is at the very core of all high performing teams (of any age.) Healthy sporting environments are places of hope and inclusion.

Covid 19 may have taught (or re-taught) many of us the true value of sport both for 'the viewer' and 'the doer'. In the early days of the pandemic in Ireland, Level 5 restrictions allowed elite-level sport to continue. My understanding is that some of the logic behind this was to give 'the viewer' something to look forward to watching at the weekend, as well as something to talk about, and think about, during the week; to give people hope and allow them feel part of something. In many ways the elite sportsperson increasingly became the modern-day gladiator; there to entertain the people and add colour and hope to their 'new normal'.

Level 5 restrictions also allowed for non-contact underage sports training to continue. In the midst of a global pandemic, our government appreciated and acknowledged the value of sport for both 'the viewer' and 'the doer'. Sport could build hope and drive a feeling of inclusion; essential for the health and wellbeing of the people.

In this piece I will write about sport for 'the doer.' Sport 'of the people, for the people and by the people.' I will talk to the sport I am involved in… 'ordinary sport'…as with everything- the ordinary can be extraordinary. I will write to You, the millennial generation, who are without doubt our next generation of 'ordinary coaches.' I too am an 'ordinary coach.'

For one reason or another, some of you may soon be coming to the end of your playing days, however, you are the generation that holds the future of sport in your hands. In this piece I will speak to the potential of 'ordinary sport' to foster hope and cultivate inclusion; to nurture the mental health of people and society. I will examine the integral role the 'ordinary coach' must assume if sports potential for good is to be realised into the future. I will challenge you; I will call you to service. I understand my chapter may be a little different to others in this book in that I will be challenging you to help others. Sport, and by extension the world, needs the best version of you.

So what is the value of 'ordinary sport' and what is the power of the 'ordinary coach'? How can sport foster hope and cultivate inclusion? How can it help the mental health of our (young) people? What does sport and coaching offer society and are we maximising their potential for good?

It is said that the coach needs the athlete, but the athlete doesn't necessarily need the coach. This, of course, is technically true, but I feel increasingly in today's society, and indeed into the future, the 'ordinary coach' holds the key to unlocking the extraordinary potential of 'ordinary sport'. After all, the coach is the one who curates and cultivates the conditions which allows the good stuff to happen: hope, inclusion and so on. I want to raise your awareness of the power, potential and scope for the 'ordinary coach' to do extraordinary good. I want to challenge you to help others.

> *'Through others we become ourselves.'*
>
> —Lev Vygotsky

Sport, at its most morally praiseworthy, is a place of human endeavour. It is a place where learning and development comes about through challenge. Sport is a place to explore the limits of human potential and to maximise what we have been given. At its most moving and noble, sport doesn't have to involve cups, medals and money. It can, and must, provide the opportunity to both exhibit and develop great moral courage, to find: enjoyment, hope, connection and meaning. Those with influence in sport hold significant societal sway. The coach is a custodian. This is a tall challenge! Traditional wisdom tells us that being involved in sport is of merit to our youth, but how can we truly harness and maximise its scope for positive?

In order to realise its potential for good I feel sport must offer a place for everyone: from the elite to the recreational, from the gifted to the not so gifted. It must be a place of inclusion; it must offer hope and a sense of belonging to everyone. Sport is not just for the talented, the champions and the early developers. 'Ordinary sport' must be for everyone and from this environment the individual will emerge to find their level if coached appropriately.

If a coach, club or team is not affording its young members adequate game-time it is fundamentally failing in its primary purpose of being a place for members of its community to play the sport in question and to encourage hope for players and participants. Yes, I appreciate the challenges involved in this, but 'the way' becomes much clearer if we understand our 'why'.

Sport is for everyone, especially so 'ordinary sport' provided the 'ordinary coach' is strong enough to lead the way, and unlock its potential. Sport can be the antidote for many of society's ills: obesity, mental health issues and addiction. Sport provides endless opportunity, and opportunity is the mother of all learning and development. For me, the primary role of sport is to teach young people lessons for life:

'Try your best, learn as you go, improvement comes through challenge and application, stick together, serve your team and teammates, learn how to win and lose with dignity... hope for better days and appreciate there will be setbacks along the way.'

Sport should be a vehicle to help people 'get better' at life, develop themselves and strengthen their constitution for this world.

When the learner is guided properly, sport affords them the opportunity to develop: mental and physical resilience, character, communication and teamwork skills, as well as leadership qualities. It provides them with a place where they feel like they belong; inclusion. This all sounds idyllic; however, the reality can often be the opposite when the leadership is weak or incompetent and example that is set is poor.

Sport can, all too often, be about the negatives of: elitism, favouritism, aggressive and disrespectful behaviour, abusive coaches and supporters and so on. I know this because at one time or another, I was either part of that, or at least a relatively willing bystander. Perhaps occasionally, I still am; passion can lead us astray.

As coaches and leaders it is our responsibility and challenge to lead with nobility and help illicit the true value of sport. This is a big order! Yes, we need to be experts in our game (clearly the technical and the tactical elements of coaching are extremely important if we expect to retain the young sportsperson) but we also need to be experts in leading by example, showing the way and educating those in our care. Sport needs us!

As coaches we must help our athletes establish: why they play, how they want to prepare, how they wish represent themselves, their team and their club, what sport can offer them and what sport means to them? Their motives will anchor their strength and drive their passion. We must provide an environment that protects the weak, challenges the strong and ensures our athletes are treated with respect, afforded opportunity and challenged appropriately. We must create a climate where the athlete is allowed to express themselves, to extend themselves and to evolve their own style and personality. To quote 'The Coaches Coach' Liam Moggan,

"If future generations are to be liberated and to thank us, we need to feed their passion and enthusiasm, and integrate fun and enjoyment into the wonderful world of sport. We need to encourage people to do something they enjoy, rather than be better at doing something than someone else".

'Sport for the viewer' must never become more important than 'sport for the doer' and our challenge as 'ordinary coaches' is to maximise sport's potential for good by recruiting and retaining as many 'doers' as possible. Healthy sporting environments are places of hope and inclusion; they are places that support the positive development of people and their mental health. Healthy sporting environments depend on strong leadership. We, 'the ordinary coach' hold great sway. We can give so much and indeed we can get so much…one of life's great symmetries… 'for it is in giving that we receive.'

I wish you well Coach.

Take Away Nuggets

- You, the millennial generation, are our next generation of sports coaches.
- Sport has the potential to give people hope, improve their mental and physical health and make them feel like they belong.
- The coach is a custodian for all that is good in sport and as so plays a key role in maximising it's potential for societal betterment.
- This world needs good sports coaches that can provide athletes with healthy sporting environments.
- 'For it is in giving we receive.'

And I think to myself… What a wonderful world.

Paul Kilgannon

Coming From A Place of Hope

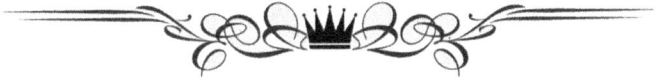

Áine Crosse

L ife has a way of knocking us down, bringing us to places we never thought we would be or ever have to face, especially when it comes to those closest to us. With me, it was my children. I had the same dreams of life that we all have, getting married, having children, living what we all like to call 'the dream'. In a heartbeat, that was all taken from us when our children were diagnosed with serious, life-changing illnesses. It started with one child and then became three. It was a diagnosis that would break our hearts. An incurable set of disorders grouped under the umbrella name of Mitochondrial Disease. A name that we were going to know inside out because it has taken over our lives. You feel like life has knocked you down, like a heavy brick hitting you over the head, but this wasn't a brick, it was much, much more.

Your life is taken over by illness, autism, hospitals. You feel like wondering, is there a light at the end of the tunnel or where is this going to end? You get lost deep inside a world of uncertainty and it becomes fight or flight with you. A decision needs to be made. Will you let this define your life, who you are, or who your children might or will become?

I decided to fight and not let this illness take over our lives in a way that destroyed us. I believed strongly that we could get through this. So our journey began, with test after test endlessly keeping the faith no matter what came our way. We were finding hope in a world where we, all too often, felt there was none.

Our journey began on the 10th of May 2006, when our son Darragh was born. He was beautiful, just perfect. At six weeks old he was sitting in his chair very quiet and he began to look very yellow. My instinct was to just leave and bring him to a doctor, and my instinct ended up being correct. Darragh had a kidney infection. I was sent straight to the hospital with him, at which time he became very ill. That was the day our lives were to change forever.

Darragh was to undergo many tests, to see if there was an underlying issue that caused his kidney infection. The specialist in the hospital told us to christen him, as they were not sure what was wrong with him, but they knew he was very ill. Our hearts sank, we felt like our world came crashing down.

It was to take another four years before we were to get a complete diagnosis for Darragh and, by this time, we had another son Sean. I was also pregnant with our daughter, Lisa during this time. We were brought back into the hospital for Darragh's results. They sat us down; the doctor held his head in his hands as he looked at us and said Darragh had a genetic condition called Mitochondrial Disease. It affects the brain, heart, kidneys, muscles and the liver we were told. "There was no cure." All we could do was look at one another, because we didn't know what it was, or why people were apologising to us, giving us a look of sympathy. We were told to go home and Google it.

Here we were home, with a diagnosis, a word, "Mitochondria." A word which meant nothing to us, one we didn't understand, but it was a word that was going to turn our lives upside down, inside out and change us forever.

As we Googled it, we discovered that this was a life -threatening disease, that would affect all of our children. So, we ended up getting Sean and Lisa tested. We were then to be informed that our three children had Mitochondrial disease, and while this was all happening, all three of our children were also diagnosed with Autism. The Autism and Mitochondrial Disease were to get worse with each child, as our youngest daughter was to be diagnosed with severe Autism. She is nonverbal, and suffers with complete meltdowns. As you can see, from what I stated at the start of this chapter, our lives were to become severely challenging, and very hard. On every level. But we swore to never give up.

Mitochondrial Disease: A life-long, life-threatening condition

So here we are, parents of children. Seven of them now. And our love for them is boundless. And yet I add a cautionary note, and it's this: you'll find guilt in endless places, and you'll find ways to carry it with you. Your love and your hope do not absolve that grief. So, too, there is a great deal of false positivity in the world; a self-betraying effort to pretend that you could never change a thing. This won't serve you in the way that you think.

Instead, perspective, is how we cope. You are allowed to say that you wish things had gone differently – scream it if you have to. Denying this won't make you a better person, and it won't bring you any measure of lasting good. The truth of it is, that ours is a heavy-handed struggle, and in it, we carve out for ourselves a path of acceptance; one that offers light; one that offers growth and sleep-filled nights and happy moments with loved ones in spite of it all. We move forward with faith in our abilities as people to adapt and overcome the many, many challenges that daily come our way.

We acknowledge that life is a double-sided coin - always turning. Happiness, just as it is with sadness, isn't made to last. One inevitably replaces the other, teaching us meaning and appreciation, and so we cherish the good days, and we learn on the bad ones. In this, we know that whatever lies ahead will be a result of our best human effort – and that we will have done it together.

For those of you in this same struggle – concern yourself less with what you're supposed to be. There are times when you have to fight tooth-and-nail and demand the extraordinary. Have courage. So, too, will there be times when the future is a terrifying thought that waits for you at the beginning of every new day. Know that there is a road through it. Know that there is hope.

Take Away Nuggets for Millennials

For me, finding out about Autism and Mitochondria was like going through some stages of grief. First, it was;

Sadness, I felt a sense of loss for the child I felt I should have had, the one that would have an ordinary life, be happy and do things that all children their age did. But then it occurred to me, why be sad? I have my child, he still has a life to live, and happiness is not about whether he's autistic or sick, it's about raising him the same as his siblings, in a happy environment.

Then came;

Blame, you feel you are to blame, you feel in a sense that it's all your fault, but it's not. It's just one of life's mysteries, of why this happened.

To me, it's my path, it may not have been what I wanted or would've chosen, but every time I see my child reach a new milestone and the smile on his face, I know this path chose me.

Then came;

Guilt, guilt was a big one for me, was it something I did wrong? But on that I discovered there was no reason to feel guilty, I didn't do anything wrong, I did all the right things during my pregnancy. This is your child's path and one you just have to walk with them, no amount of guilt is ever going to change that.

Last but not least, the most important one;

Acceptance, I know it's one of the hardest things to do, is to accept that this happened to your child and in your life, but I really feel that no matter how hard it feels to do this, if you cannot accept what happened then how can you ask others to accept it? We as parents always put out there that we want acceptance for Autism, for our children. But at the end of the day, that acceptance needs to start with us. If we don't feel it inside, how can we expect the outside world to. So, no matter how much your life has changed, which it has, there's no point in saying any different, acceptance will always be the key for you as a parent, and for your beautiful child in moving forward.

On Escaping Being a Hostage to Expectation

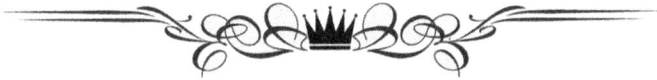

Anna Gray

"I know that I'm a prisoner to all my father held so dear, I know that I'm a hostage to all his hopes and fears"

—Mike & The Mechanics - The Living Years.

I'm not sure my hopes for my life were ever truly my own when I was a child. Looking back now, I can see how they were a combination of parents, siblings, teachers and perhaps a little of mine. Looking back, I think I absorbed many of the ideas of what other people thought I should end up doing with my life and of what they hoped would happen for me.

My parents weren't born into an area of Belfast that really promoted education. Northern Ireland in the 1960s, when they would have been attending school, was more focussed on the strife in the streets than on educating the population. They had to really fight for their education, really try, really step out of the norm here. They had to really want to better themselves as there were so many things against them. Poverty was very real here, and surviving was the main objective.

My Dad was the only person in his whole school that year to pass his 11+, that's one person out of at least 50. He was the only one of his entire friends or family circle to go to university and get a good job. He did that for himself. He had so many hopes for his life, and he wanted something better than what was on offer in the streets of Belfast. I'm extremely proud of him. He became a teacher and a writer himself and the choices he made meant that we got to be a family who could invest time and energy in education.

Sadly, my Mum wasn't granted the same opportunities. She came from a large family and there was plenty of housework to be done and things that needed mending and younger siblings to feed. She never got the chance to formally educate herself as her own schoolwork came last in a long line of things she was given to help out with. She passed away last year and it's one thing she would often bring up. She would say that she wondered how different things would have been on a career level for her if she had more chances in school. She had an amazing artistic ability that she expressed in many ways over the years. I only wish she had received more recognition for it.

Both my parents had high hopes for their children, like any parent would. I remember feeling like I just wanted to make them proud. My Dad had three brothers, all of whom were very intelligent and in excellent jobs. I wanted to be like them, to speak the way that they did and be interesting like they seemed to be. I didn't really leave any room for my own gifts to shine through, I simply wanted to be like them and to do the things that they did. That was a mistake. That led me to ignore who I was and to simply try to replicate their life choices.

It's interesting, I'm discovering as I'm writing this, that this is the sacrifice, I silently made in order to be more accepted and loved. I took on the hopes of other people and tried to realise them in my own life, to please them, to be celebrated, to be part of the tribe. Nobody said I had to do that. I did it without even knowing what I was doing, until years later.

One day I overheard my parents say how delighted they were that I wanted to study Law. I was far too young (maybe 8 or 9) to be making choices or steps that would bind me to it, but I certainly thought that's what I wanted to do. Their happiness filled me with a sense of belonging, I knew they hoped I would pick something along those lines. They wanted me to have what they viewed as a good and stable career. To be entirely honest, I only thought I would like to do it because it looked great on TV, glamourous and, somehow, intellectual. I had no comprehension of what was really involved.

As life went by, I felt lost and torn. Torn between what I thought I should be doing and what I was learning about myself and what I was good at. They didn't seem to match up. I was finding out that I wasn't so much of an intellectual, I was more drawn to being with people, listening to them, finding out how they worked. I wanted to learn about nutrition, body health, mind, body, spirit stuff and angels. Stuff that there were no real jobs in, no money in, no security in - or so I thought.

When it came time for me to choose my A-level subjects that would lead to my degree course, I panicked. I chose subjects I didn't feel passionate about. I chose what I thought I should choose for stability and approval, ending up choosing a degree in English Literature. Whilst that would be great for a lot of people, it wasn't the right choice for me.

I was the only one in my family who ever dropped out of university. I left after a year and few months. I rarely turned up for lectures and my work was always below average and late – not because I wasn't intelligent or because I was careless – I simply didn't enjoy it and found it impossible to put so much of myself into something that I disliked so much.

On the one hand, I felt massive relief, on the other a loss of hope and an overwhelming sense of failure.

I had no idea of how to move forward with my life, what I wanted to do or how to deal with feeling that I had failed. There was no pressure put on me by my family, they just wanted me to be happy, but I somehow felt that I wasn't part of the tribe anymore, that I had excluded myself from the 'club'. I knew it wasn't what they had hoped for me and that made it worse.

Somewhere inside me I still had high hopes for my future, I still wanted to study, to grow and to learn – I just didn't know in what area yet. I spent the next few years in jobs I didn't like, struggling to find my path forward. I had a daughter at 23 years old and suddenly studying again was not an option, or at least wouldn't be for quite some time. So, there I was, a university drop out and a single parent. All the things I had never wanted to be, all the things I had feared meant the end of any career prospects. And to be honest, it really did limit my prospects at the time.

Something amazing happened though, through dropping out and feeling like a failure, I learned humility. Through having a child, I learned very quickly about deep love and connection. I think those were two lessons that I really needed to learn to prepare myself for a different kind of life, one that I could live from the heart, with authenticity.

When my daughter turned four, I began to study again, this time I knew exactly what I wanted to do. I knew I wanted to help others who had experienced similar difficulties to my own. I began a counselling course, one that would eventually lead me to be able to work with clients. I also studied psychotherapy, gestalt therapy, grief counselling and substance abuse counselling. It would take around 5 years before I would be able to work with people, but I had found what I loved and what felt right for me to be dedicating myself to.

What I had perceived as my failures, turned out to be the things that helped me to understand who I really was and in what direction I wanted to go. When I stopped taking on the hopes of others as my own, and really learned who I was as a person, that's when my life started to work.

The quote that I opened this chapter with always rings in my head. I often see how some of us feel we must live out the hopes and dreams of previous generations in order to be loved and accepted by them, we must somehow follow in their footsteps. This can occur, as it did with me, with no pressure from them, no vocalised expectations, but rather a subtle unspoken something that happens inside that is really quite powerful and potentially damaging.

Or, it can be outright and obvious, where we are told we must do this, or that, or live in a certain way in order to be somehow 'included' in the family circle.

Either way, the results can be that we end up choosing what others hope for us over what we hope for ourselves, and that rarely turns out well. I thought I had failed in the eyes of my family and myself simply because my path was different to theirs. It was different to that of my siblings. What I had hoped for myself at that young age, to become a lawyer and impress all my family with my fantastic intellectualism, hadn't worked out. Picking a degree in something I didn't enjoy, hadn't worked out. Trying to please others even when they didn't ask me to, hadn't worked out.

The only thing that did work out, was learning that everybody is different, our paths won't all look the same, there isn't one straight path to personal success. We can have a hundred different hopes for our futures, and they might not end up coming to fruition - that doesn't mean we are failures. I learned that it was ok to 'fail' and to try and try again. I always say some of the most interesting people I've ever met, don't know what they want to do with their lives, even when they are in their thirties or forties. I found that when I lived from a place of deep authenticity, I was at my happiest. It's not always as easy as it sounds to do that, there can be mental and emotional barriers to push through to get there. We can often feel we are letting other people down; we can sometimes feel as if we need the permission of other people to live our own truth. Sometimes, everything we try just simply doesn't work, because we are doing it to please other people, so we can end up with no choice left but to put ourselves first, to do the scary thing, to take the risk of being judged or ridiculed for the sake of our own happiness.

It's worth it, and the sooner we can get there, the sooner our lives can feel like our own without the burdens of trying to be something other than what we are. In the end, my life is very different from what I had expected in my earlier years, but it's more than I could have hoped for.

Take Away Nuggets

1. I would encourage very honest discussions with parents, teachers and anyone else who holds a significant place in your circle about what you really want to do with your life. That little voice inside can quickly turn into a shout if it isn't expressed.
2. It can really help to understand your family background and how that may have impacted your parents/guardians hopes for you, especially if they are different from your own.
3. You can only live your life, not anyone else's. You are the one who must get up every day and do whatever it is you have chosen to do. Make it something you can bear, or even better, something that you absolutely love. Don't be a prisoner to anyone else's hopes and fears.

Hope for an Industry in Crisis

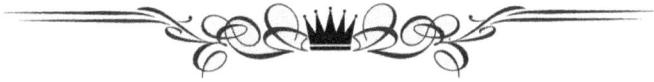

Jennifer Murphy

Introduction

Having worked in Human Resources within the Hospitality sector for almost a decade, I have witnessed first-hand, the many challenges presented to the industry and have been humbled at how leaders in this sector remain resilient. While there is no doubt, that many businesses in the grip of the COVID-19 pandemic struggled to remain viable, it seems to me that the Irish Hospitality industry was practically brought to its knees.

The industry which, in Ireland, ordinarily contributes in the region of €5 - €7.6 billion to the economy (Deloitte, 2021), and primarily the livelihoods of its precarious atypical workers, who are strongly represented in this sector, were all but decimated. In the grip of a global and national emergency, the decisions made by those in Government, regardless of one's individual opinion, ultimately faced a Sisyphean struggle to protect public health whilst attempting to prevent an economic crisis. It is arguable that whilst flattening the curve, the measures simultaneously flattened the

Hospitality industry. What follows, is an overview of the impact of the COVID-19 pandemic, within this sector through the lens of Talent Acquisition and Talent Management.

Most people in Ireland will vividly recall the events of the first quarter of 2020, where the first whispers of an outbreak of a virus in China soon turned to widespread panic and fear as SARS-CoV-2 or Coronavirus spread uncontrollably throughout the world. As the world looked on in fear and disbelief, hospitals quickly became overwhelmed, case numbers rose at an inconceivable velocity, and subsequently, the unbearable collective pain for the people and families behind the alarming mortality rates was a very grim reality.

In every country, unprecedented measures were implemented to slow the spread of this deadly virus and, in Ireland, following weeks of multiple cancellations of public events, on March 17th, 2020, in order to protect the healthcare system and to prevent the spread of the virus within the population, it was formally announced that Ireland would move into lockdown for an initial period of two weeks.

Closure

Closures of all businesses with the exception of "essential retail" was deemed necessary and mandatory. Employers were advised, where possible, that staff should work from home or alternatively be temporarily laid off. Unsurprisingly, the vast majority of Hospitality workers cannot perform their work remotely, therefore suffered an acute and sudden loss of income without any indication as to the duration of the uncertainty they faced. Disconnected from their place of work, shut off from colleagues and all social aspects of being part of a team, in an industry which prides itself on providing guest service and being around people, loneliness and anxiety were commonly reported to Human Resources teams.

For those fortunate enough to remain in employment, an extreme level of adaptability had to be deployed to sustain the mental strength and focus to perform both professionally and survive personally. Leaders within the sector had to find deeper levels of resourcefulness and grit to navigate not only a global health crisis, but also, a seemingly unyielding economic war against multiple closures, rising costs, furloughed teams, recruitment challenges, tarnished industry reputation as a result of continuous and often disproportionately negative media coverage and the tidal wave of anxiety and mental health issues which dominated the agenda once a return to work became possible. Some two years later, as the industry limps from the COVID-19 battlefield, we look to hope, for recovery for the sector and its people.

Human Resource Practitioners in this sector, might posit, is recovery possible and can Hospitality ever aspire to become an industry of choice for top talent? Pre-pandemic, Hospitality has been broadly understood to be less favourable than most industries due to multiple factors including, its reputation for lagging the market in terms of remuncration, lack of any additional benefits namely healthcare, pensions, additional annual leave to name but a few. Depending on the size of a property and facilities within, for those in operational or entry level positions, more often than not, minimum wage and a staff meal is often all that is available to attract candidates.

The Great Resignation

For those in middle management, the standard salary packages available often fall short of those offered in comparable roles within other similar tertiary industries. In the aftermath of "The Great Resignation" Human Resource leaders now have a serious challenge ahead, to stem the flow of employees exiting the sector and to utilise this talent crisis as a platform to turn the perception of Hospitality as a "stop gap job" into a fulfilling career. Never before has there been such an opportunity to reset and restart. However, of all the learnings we can take from the impact of COVID-19, one thing is acutely apparent - leaders of Hospitality organisations have a responsibility to not only reassess the approach to Talent Management but must accept, that a change in attitude is a fundamental requirement if the industry is to claw its way back from the abyss. To build strength in one's team, it is imperative to understand what your people want, management must listen, respond and be consistent. The time for "old school" style leadership has long since passed and is beyond abhorrent to the woke generation.

Hospitality industry leaders have a responsibility to not only create decent standards of employment for the current labour force but a duty of care for the protection of the industry into the future. What millennials and Gen-Z workers want, has been much publicised and researched and I have written about this elsewhere (Murphy, 2021) as have colleagues in this book (Callanan and McKenna, 2021; MacGiolla Bhuí, 2021; Noone; 2021).

Hospitality leaders must be cognisant of the difference between relational and transactional reward (De Smet, 2021). The millennial and Gen-Z want flexibility, work-life balance, meaningful work and fulfilment and they will simply not stay where this is not provided as shown in the much-publicised work of "The Great Resignation", which demonstrated the willingness of employees to leave their role even without having another position secured in advance. These momentous decisions leave Hospitality in a very precarious position.

In June 2021, Hospitality reopened the doors to leisure guests after what was the longest closure in Ireland to date, during the COVID-19 pandemic. Depending on location, some properties struggled to maintain a basic occupancy for the remainder of the year yet, conversely others, generally in a more rural setting, experienced unprecedented levels of business (IHF 2021) as the domestic leisure market boomed and people could not get out of their lockdown lives fast enough. The guest was back, and they had serious expectations, and rightly so. Price increases were apparent as hotels worked hard to offset the expense of providing extensive safety measures for staff and guests and to counteract the impact of multiple closures. In the midst of a whirlwind, transitioning from complete closure to sudden full occupancy levels, hiring managers, recruiters and talent acquisition professionals found themselves navigating a barren landscape struggling to place candidates at all levels of the organisation and the trend continues to the present day with over 40,000 hospitality vacancies recently reported (Failte Ireland,2022).

Among HR professionals, the true figure is believed to be much higher as it is not possible to accurately reflect the level of ghost turnover within properties, whereby employees are disengaged, and actively looking for a new role but have not yet physically resigned. Human Resource teams reported increased levels of stress, anxiety and overwhelm as teams were catapulted from the safety and calm of their homes into a familiar but very different workplace (Rosenberg et al,2021) and (AlMala, 2020). For middle and senior management, the unprecedented levels of emotional labour, combined with the demands of a management role created the perfect storm for burnout, the prelude to walk out.

The Law of Attraction

Although it may seem obvious to suggest the perceived safety of a work environment has an impact on the employees' level of security, both physical and psychological. Nevertheless, research has shown that employees who feel safe in their workplace, are much less likely to harbour turnover intent. Aside from the statutory requirement to protect one's employees, it is reasonable for an employee to expect this level of safeguarding from an employer as standard. However, during the COVID-19 pandemic when return to work was imminent, employers were required to reassess every area and implement additional and often extreme safety measures which, paradoxically, had the effect of simultaneously increasing levels of anxiety and frustration (Mao et al, 2020) as staff returned to a familiar building with very different control measures in place. Chinazzi et al (2020) compare the risk factors between the role of front-line Hospitality workers to that of front-line medical staff, both share exposure to high volumes of people within a pressurised, fast paced environment. Often working long hours to compensate for the absence of other team members who have fallen victim to the rapidly spreading, highly infectious, potentially life threating disease, thus, naturally, anxiety levels began to rise within organisations. This issue was further compounded for workers in closer contact roles such as Spa Therapists, conducting deeply personal work with guests and also for workers in mandatory quarantine properties where the potential for infection was heightened. For many, the mandatory face mask provided not only a safety shield. but also, a veil to conceal the anxiety as workers were reminded to "smile with your eyes" a now famous term in hospitality pandemic customer service training. As previously stated, atypical workers, characterised as casual, fixed term or temporary workers, represent a large proportion of the hospitality labour force. They are by their very nature, precarious workers and generally receive little more than minimum wage for their efforts. Suffice to say the emotional labour and relentless demands placed on this cohort during the various waves of the pandemic were all too often overwhelming and beyond endurance.

As the country moved through various waves, mutations of the disease, lockdowns, reopening's, constant government "leaked" announcements and continuous negativity in the media, employee anxiety levels rising faster than the reported daily case numbers, the Hospitality industry took a battering like no other. This meant that the ability to retain teams, whilst attempting to keep engagement and morale levels up, was a near impossible task. Employee psychological capital was tested to its limits. Luthans et al (2002) describe human psychological capital as the ability to adapt and remain resilient, optimistic and hopeful in situations of stress, it is the state which drives employee behaviour. Organisations who carefully implement safeguarding policies, lead with authenticity, congruence and consistency, who have robust corporate social responsibility policies, and comprehensive employee wellbeing programmes are best placed to successfully weather the storm and retain employees. The aforementioned all contribute to an overarching perception of genuine care and trust, which in turn, leads to increased levels of employee optimism, enhanced ability to cope in crisis and reduce the duration of recovery when anxiety spikes (Mao 2020).

Wen et al (2018) show that there are always multiple factors involved in the employee's decision to exit the organisation, these include, but are not limited to; age, gender, family status and family responsibility, financial constraints and commitments. What Millennial and Gen Z workers want and expect from employers is much publicised and researched. What is known, is that this cohort require a more holistic employment experience therefore, salary and benefits only form part of what is considered attractive. Millennials want work life balance, additional annual leave, reduced working hours, development and progression, flexibility to work remotely or hybrid within an organisation which prioritises sustainability, inclusion and wellbeing. The delineation of the advantages of a career in Hospitality at recruitment stage is imperative to attract candidates, and, furthermore, the onboarding and assimilation period must be fully congruent throughout.

A Need for Sector Transformation

The incorporation of the aforementioned, requires a transformation within the sector, albeit arguably, a necessity if Hospitality leaders wish to ameliorate the current perception of Hospitality as a credible career for top talent. Recent changes in legislation will provide for some of the work life balance the post Covid-19 employee craves, such as extended parents leave and the introduction of mandatory sick pay from 2022, proposals to allow workers the right to request hybrid and remote working arrangements. For more senior positions, the right to disconnect is certainly a game-changer for the boss who struggles with boundaries, as shown in the ground-breaking Kepak case (Kepak V O'Hara, Labour Court, 2018). Ms. O'Hara was employed as a Business Development Executive for Kepak Convenience Foods, based in Blanchardstown, Dublin and was contracted to work 40 hours per week. Ms O'Hara's role involved travelling to other customer sites in Leinster which took a considerable amount of her time. Her manager complained that her weekly reporting was slower than the company expected, and an improvement was required. Following the feedback, Ms. O'Hara felt obliged to continue to work after her contracted hours to fulfil her reporting and administrative duties. In April 2017, the employment relationship between both parties ended, and a complaint was lodged by Ms O'Hara to the Workplace Relations Commission under the Organisation of Working Time Act 1997. Evidence was submitted to support the fact that the complainant had worked in her own time, including early mornings, late evenings and weekends to meet the demands of her workload. Emails were also submitted as evidence that Ms. O'Hara had regularly worked up to sixty hours per week. The Adjudicating officer determined that Kepak had infringed upon section 15 of The Organisation of Working Time Act with regards to the employee working in excess of a 48-hour week, the statutory maximum set out in the legislation. Ms O'Hara was awarded €7,500 in compensation, however the president set by this decision sent shockwaves to many organisations. Hospitality now faces an even greater challenge than lockdown, as the industry needs to adapt once more to become attractive to career driven Millennials. Notwithstanding, there is a great opportunity to pivot and recuperate from the recent crisis and shine a light on Hospitality careers.

References

Akgunduz, Y., Eryilmaz, G., 2018. Does turnover intention mediate the effects of job insecurity and co-worker support on social loafing? Int. J. Hosp. Manag. 68, 41–49. https://doi.org/10.1016/j.ijhm.2017.09.010.

AlMala, Wassim, How COVID-19 Changes the HRM Practices (Adapting One HR Strategy May Not Fit to All) (November 24, 2020). Available at SSRN: https://ssrn.com/abstract=3736719 or http://dx.doi.org/10.2139/ssrn.3736719

Bjorklund, C., 2007. Work motivation and perceived risks. Int. J. Risk Assess. Manag. 7 (2), 237–247. https://doi.org/10.1504/IJRAM.2007.011734

Chen, H., Ayoun, B., Eyoun, K., 2018. Work-family conflict and turnover intentions: a study comparing China and U.S. hotel employees. J. Hum. Resour. Hosp. Tour. 17 (2), 247–269. https://doi.org/10.1080/15332845.2017.1406272.

Chinazzi, M., Davis, T.J., Ajelli, M., Gioannini, C., Litvinova, M., Merler, S., et al., 2020. The effect of travel restrictions on the spread of the 2019 novel coronavirus (COVID19) outbreak. Science 368 (6489), 395–400. https://doi.org/10.1126/science. aba9757

De Witte, H., 1999. Job insecurity and psychological well-being: review of the literature and exploration of some unresolved issues. Eur. J. Work. Organ. Psychol. 8 (2), 155–177. https://doi.org/10.1080/135943299398302.

DeJoy, D.M., Schaffer, B.S., Wilson, M.G., Vandenberg, R.J., Butts, M.M., 2004. Creating safer workplaces: assessing the determinants and role of safety climate. J. Safety Res. 35 (1), 81–90. https://doi.org/10.1016/j.jsr.2003.09.018.

Herscovitch, L., Meyer, J.P., 2002. Commitment to organizational change: extension of a three-component model. J. Appl. Psychol. 87 (3), 474–487. https://doi.org/ 10.1037/0021-9010.87.3.474.

Kim, J., 2018. The contrary effects of intrinsic and extrinsic motivation on burnout and turnover intention in the public sector. Int. J. Manpow. 39 (3), 486–500. https://doi. org/10.1108/IJM-03-2017-0053.

Kim, Y.G., Kim, S., Yoo, J.L., 2012. Travel agency employees' career commitment and turnover intention during the recent global economic crisis.

Serv. Ind. J. 32 (8), 1247–1264. https://doi.org/10.1080/02642069.2010.545393.

Lee, S.H., Jeong, D.Y., 2017. Job insecurity and turnover intention: organizational commitment as mediator. Soc. Behav. Pers. 45 (4), 529–536. https://doi.org/ 10.2224/sbp.5865.

Mao, Y., He, J., Morrison, A.M., Coca-Stefaniak, J.A., 2020. Effects of tourism CSR on employee psychological capital in the COVID-19 crisis: from the perspective of conservation of resources theory. Curr. Issues Tourism. https://doi.org/10.1080/ 13683500.2020.1770706.

Martins, A., Riordan, T., Dolnicar, S., 2020. A post-COVID-19 model of tourism and hospitality workforce resilience. SocArXiv. https://doi.org/10.31235/osf.io/4quga.

Opatha,H (2020). "The Coronavirus and The Employees: A Study from the Point of Human Resource Management Article". Sri LankanJournal of Human ResourceManagement,38,39

Rosenberg,A, Adams,M, Polick, Li,W, Dang, J &Hsin-Chun J Tsai (2021) COVID-19 and mental health of food retail, food service, and hospitality workers, Journal of Occupational and Environmental Hygiene, 18:4-5, 169-179, DOI: 10.1080/15459624.2021.1901905

Ryan, R.M., Deci, E.L., 2000. Self-determination theory and the facilitation of intrinsic motivation, social development, and well-being. Am. Psychol. 55 (1), 68–78. https://doi.org/10.1037/0003-066X.55.1.68.

Smith, T.D., 2018. An assessment of safety climate, job satisfaction and turnover intention relationships using a national sample of workers from the United States. Int. J. Occup. Saf. Ergon. 24 (1), 27–34. https://doi.org/10.1080/ 10803548.2016.1268446.

Wen, T., Zhang, Y., Wang, X., Tang, G., 2018. Factors influencing turnover intention among primary care doctors: a crosssectional study in Chongqing, China. Human Resour. Health 16, 10. https://doi.org/10.1186/s12960-018-0274-z.

Zhou, Q., Lai, X., Wan, C., Zhang, X., Tan, L., 2020. Prevalence and impact of burnout, secondary traumatic stress and compassion satisfaction on hand hygiene of healthcare workers in medical aid team during COVID-19 pandemic. Res. Square. https://doi.org/10.21203/rs.3.rs-28820/v1

Reports

Failte Ireland Hotel Sector Review, Spring 2022

Deloitte Hospitality, Tourism Sector Domestic Market Review 2021

Websites

https://www.workplacerelations.ie/en/cases/2018/july/dwt1820.html [accessed March 13 2022]

https://www.thejournal.ie/recruitment-crisis-hospitality-sector-5676742-Feb2022 [accessed Feb 19 2022]

https://www.independent.ie/irish-news/tourism-recovery-at-risk-as-40000-jobs-go-unfilled-41306862.html [accessed Feb 3rd 2022]

Legislation

Organisation of Working Time Act, 1997

Parent's Leave and Benefit Act 2019

The Safety, Health and Welfare at Work Act, 2005

Employment (Miscellaneous Provisions) Act, 2018

Terms of Employment (Information) Acts, 1994 to 2014

It's A Kind Of Magic

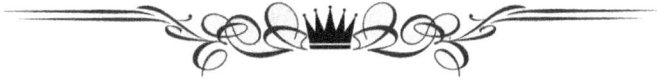

Giselle Marrinan MSc

"All the flowers of all the tomorrows are in the seeds of today."
—Chinese *Proverb*

Let Nature Teach Us

Every time I plant seeds in Autumn, I am reminded of the hope I place in this simple task. The expectation that the flowers will peep through in Spring because of my action. I have done my job and nature will do the rest, under the surface of the cold, dark, damp soil. The seeds know that when the days get a little longer and the temperature starts to rise, that it is time to reach from the darkness into the light. No one tells them to do this, but as if by magic, they know when the time is right. Incidentally a cherry tree can wait for a hundred years to grow ("Lab Girl" Hope Jahren, 2016). So it is with most seeds, it's not *if* they will grow but *when*. Witnessing my seeds flourish in Spring, gives me hope of warmer weather, long halcyon evenings and days spent at the beach. Like the flowers, my energy rises and my smile gets wider. It's like a rebirth of the spirit, soul and body.

Similarly, the butterfly beautifully symbolises hope. It begins life in one form and transforms into another protected by its cocoon while in transition. It starts off life as a crawler and metamorphoses into a magnificent flying insect. In the Christian faith, butterflies, represent death and resurrection.

In 'Hope for the Flowers' (Paulus 1972), there is a beautiful line which goes "Tell me sir, what is a butterfly?" "It's what you are meant to become. It flies with beautiful wings and joins the earth to heaven. It drinks only nectar from the flowers and carries the seeds of love from one flower to another."

There Is an Energy Behind Hope

It is amazing how many wealthy people started out life in dire poverty and rose up to succeed against all the odds – no money, wrong postal code, and no education. What is the one thing they all have in common? Hope that their life can and will get better. Hope opens us up to possibilities.

Take, for instance, the story behind the author of "It's a Long Way from Penny Apples (2003)," Bill Cullen. He was born in a socio-economically deprived area of Dublin in the 1940s, one of 14 children. He rose to become one of Irelands most successful businessmen. His story is inspiring on so many levels. From an early age, he knew everything there was to know about selling. But one thing which stood out for me, was the belief he had in himself, that his mum instilled in him. Whilst they were watching J.F. Kennedy's inspiring speech to Dáil Éireann in, 1963, his mum turned to Bill and ruffling his hair said, "*You see. There's nothing you can't do*". This one statement lived with him all his life and inspired him to hope for a better, brighter future.

Similarly, with the designer Ralph Lauren who also had a deprived start in life, he rose to create the clothing empire which needs no introduction today. When he was a child, he loved fashion but couldn't afford to get anything new. He is quoted as saying, *"When I'd get my brothers hand-me-downs, there was an energy in me that made me say 'I want to get my own things, to make my own statement". Somewhere along the line, that energy turned into something".*

Both these men had something else in common, they knew what hope involved. People think that hope and wishful thinking are the same, but they aren't. In an article by Elaine Houston (2022) in Positive Psychology, she states

"Hope is an active process, wishing is ambiguous and passive because it does not involve a plan of how to accomplish change."

There must be agency behind one's plan. Active and passive are words at opposite ends of the scale, but there is another element needed in the mix, belief in yourself. It is the catalyst.

Tell Your Heart to Beat Again (Belief)

A few years ago, I heard this marvellous song, "Tell Your Heart to Beat Again" (Phillips, Craig and Dean 2014) which touched me deeply. Then in the last year, I heard the powerful story behind it. Apparently, a pastor in Ohio approached a heart surgeon in his parish and told him that he had always wanted to see a heart procedure for real. The surgeon invited him to an open-heart surgery as an observer from the viewing gallery. The operation went perfectly. They split open the woman's sternum, removed the heart and before placing it back in her chest cavity, restarted it. For some reason the woman flatlined and all around the theatre thought she had died. Then the surgeon knelt down beside his patient and whispered something in her ear. At that moment the heart started beating again. The pastor asked the surgeon what he had whispered into the woman's ear, and this is what he said, *"Mrs. Johnson, this is your surgeon. The operation went perfectly, your heart has been repaired, now tell your heart to beat again."*

So, what does this mean for us? We can have all the hope in the world, make a brilliant plan and move strategically towards our goal but never achieve it. Why when we took all the right steps towards it, do we sometimes fail at the last hurdle? Because perhaps we don't have enough belief in ourselves that it will work, or the faith that we are good enough to deserve it. We self-sabotage. Metaphorically, we need to tell our hearts to beat again.

Make Sure That What You Hope for Is Really What You Want (Hope + Plan, but no manifestation. Why?)

I always ask people to check in with their reality when they hope for change. We work through everything they want to see moving forward in their lives, but with one critical addition. I ask them to fast forward into their new life and see how it 'fits'. It always amazes me how many people want to make changes at this stage. So, try my exercise below (Marrinan, 2018) after you focus on your dreams and see what happens.

There is no rush with this exercise, the slower and more deliberate the steps, the better. Engage a trusted friend to read the script to you so that all you have to concentrate on, are the words and feelings.

In this example, I choose career change, but it could be reworked for any change/hope you may want to focus on for your life.

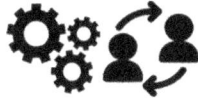

Exercise

Close your eyes if it helps to focus and imagine the following (*allow time between each step before moving onto the next one*):

1. You are day one in your new job, whether self-employed or working for a company. Or perhaps, you have decided to take time out to study for a new career...

2. Look around you; see how this new environment looks ...

3. How are you feeling inside? Are you excited? Somewhat apprehensive? Feeling more alive than you have for years...

4. If you wanted more free time, how is your life looking now? Have you more quality time with your friends and family?

5. Is this new life really motivating you and if so, how are you relating differently to people around you?

6. To make this change, have you had to make compromises and or sacrifices along the way?

7. If so, has this changed your income? How is this making you feel?

8. Has it necessitated retraining and/or returning to college?

9. Has it necessitated radical changes in lifestyle such as downsizing? If so, how is this for you?

10. How has this change been received by your loved ones? Is it the response you expected?

11. Do you feel able to press ahead with your new plans regardless of any obstacles?

12. Take a deep breath, open your eyes, and come back to the room.

Make notes on thoughts, concerns, or ideas that came up for you during this exercise, for discussion at a future date. Now, the question remains, how do I move forward with my plans? Ground your vision with a **S.M.A.R.T'** plan. This tool, first outlined by Doran (1981) is helpful in ensuring effective planning. It is a way of converting your hopes into practical, actionable goals, ensuring they have the best chance of becoming a reality.

> **Specific** – What exactly do you want to be/do in life? It isn't enough to say, I want to work in a hospital. It would be better to say, I want to be a doctor, nurse, radiographer, administrator or whatever. Being vague will not achieve your goal. Be specific.

> **Measurable**- Set incremental goals or staging posts to achieve your plan. This might necessitate up-skilling to change careers. You may want to gain an apprenticeship before moving jobs. You may have to do a business course before starting your own business.

> **Actionable**-You may want to become the CEO of a top pharmaceutical company, but you will need to get a job with them first and work your way up the ladder. I became a sales rep for the multi-national I set my sights on and worked my way expeditiously through the ranks. This way, I learnt all the different aspects of the company.

> **Realistic**-Do you have the resources and knowledge to achieve your plan? Is this the right plan for you, given your age and where you are in life? I used to play intermediate tennis in my 20s, but sadly I won't be taking on the Williams sisters at this stage in my life!

> ➢ **Timed**-Without a timeframe your plans will remain wishes. Too much time and you will lose momentum; too little time and you won't be properly prepared, and you run the risk of becoming demotivated. You may want to set out micro goals in days, weeks, months, or years. So long as you choose your timing and stick to it, you will be on track.

Have fun in the process and remember why you are doing this in the first place. Keep this foremost in your mind. It could be to have more free time with family or friends; retire early; challenge yourself; whatever it is, this will keep you motivated, when the going gets tough. Just to remind you again, make sure that what you hope for is realistic – keep grounded.

According to **Snyder's Hope Theory (1991),** hopefulness is comprised of 3 distinct but inter-related components:

1. **Goals Thinking** – The clear conceptualisation of valuable goals.
2. **Pathways Thinking** – The capacity to develop specific strategies to reach those goals.
3. **Agency Thinking** – The ability to initiate and sustain the motivation for using those strategies.

Based on these 3 components, what can we do?

Time to act!

1. So, what do I need to do now to make this hope a reality?
2. Who will be affected by these changes?
3. Who do I need to talk to first? Family, partner, boss? Have I a speech in mind?
4. How and what am I going to say and to whom? (Remember, if you need to leave your present job, it is better you speak up now rather than let it fester.)

5. Investigate the option, to cut back my hours in my present job; whilst experimenting with my new life.

6. When am I planning on making these changes? Have I a time frame?

7. There may be obstacles and if so, how will I overcome them? (As the saying goes, *'an obstacle is often a stepping stone'.*)

Hold on Tightly, Let Go Lightly

This statement, 'hold on tightly, let go lightly', came from the old Japanese Judi Sensei saying. What does it mean for us? So, we have hope for something, we have devised a plan and we have hope, but in the end it doesn't happen. This could be that it doesn't hold the magic it first held for us when we focussed on it, it wasn't realistic in the first place, or that we let obstacles come in our way, unchallenged. After weighing up the reasons, we may need to let go our grip and move on towards something else. We need to have the flexibility and optimism to create renewed hope. George Rego (2019), tells us that,

"The message is about the yin and yang balance between two ideas that seem juxtaposed to one another. The first being full commitment and the second being the flexibility to adapt and make a change"

Try not to have tunnel vision towards things. We must explore all possibilities for our lives no matter what circumstances we find ourselves in. Across the age spectrum from millennials to seniors, there is always, like a good chess player, another move.

As a bonus, a sense of hope has been found to be good for our health, even when things look gloomy. I recall the Viennese psychiatrist, Viktor Frankl's (2004), observations in the holocaust concentration camps in Germany, during WW2. He is purported to have said that, "*He who has a why to live, can bear with almost any how.*"

Faith and Spiritual Support

In my world, my faith in God keeps me going and gives me hope. I try to align my plans with what I envisage His will is for my life path. This belief helps me overcome obstacles and keeps me focussed particularly when the going gets tough. I recall the joke I heard years ago where a man says to God, "*Please God, help me win the lottery*". There is a pregnant pause, then a voice booms from the heavens, "*Do me a favour my child*, meet me halfway, buy a lottery ticket". So, you see, even with faith you must do some legwork yourself!

Word of Caution – A Time and a Place

Don't let your sense of hope take away from the present. What do I mean by this? Think about a situation where you might have been or are, caring for someone sick, even terminally ill. It is right and proper that you are holding out hope for a cure, but if all your energies are consumed in future possibilities, then you will miss out on the moments with this precious person in the NOW.

No matter what your hopes and hence your plans are for the future, remember to live in the only moment of which you are certain, the present.

> "*A rainbow is a prism that sends shards of multicoloured light in various directions. It lifts our spirits and makes us think of what is possible. Hope is the same – a personal rainbow of the mind.*"

—Charles Snyder

References

http://www.wsj.com/public/resources/documents/LABGIRL_excerpt.pdf

Paulus, T. "Hope for the Flowers"1972. Paulist Press

Cullen, B." It's a Long Way from Penny Apples" Hodder and Stoughton, 2003.

Houston, E., "What is Hope in Psychology"
https://positivepsychology.com/hope-therapy/ 2022

https://freeccm.com/2014/01/20/story-behind-the-song-with-phillips-craig-dean-tell-your-heart-to-beat-again/

Marrinan, G. "Another Zero" Book Hub Publishing 2018

Doran, G. T. (1981). "There's a S.M.A.R.T. Way to Write Management's Goals and Objectives", Management Review, Vol. 70, Issue 11, pp. 35-36.

Snyder, C. R., Irving, L. M., & Anderson, J. R. (1991). Hope and health. In C. R. Snyder & D. R. Forsyth (Eds.), Pergamon general psychology series, Vol. 162. "*Handbook of social and clinical psychology: The health perspective* "(pp. 285-305). Elmsford, NY: Pergamon Press.

Rego, G., "" Hang on Tightly Let Go Lightly" https://floridajukido.com/hang-on-tightly-let-go-lightly/ Feb 2019

Frankl, V. E., "Man's Search for Meaning" Rider. 2004

Spiralling Through Life

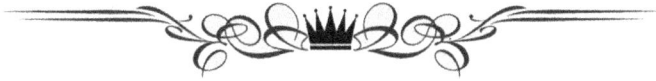

Keith Russell

Introduction

For a long period of my life I hid in the shadows, metaphorically and literally. But, not anymore. My life has completely evolved in the last 18 months. In this chapter, I'll give some insight into my story, but I also want to highlight that there can be light at the end of the tunnel, there is hope. I'm living proof of this. I've been silent for a long time about my own struggles with mental health, for multiple reasons, on which I will try to expand.

My Voice

I'm probably better known for being the creator of 'The Endless Spiral', which is a mental health podcast and blog. In a short space of time, I have been nominated for multiple awards and gained a large social media presence. But that's not what my path is all about. It's about self-improvement and helping people share their stories. I've been on somewhat of a journey recently sharing my own story of living with several mental conditions and I must admit, it has felt like an enormous weight has been lifted from my shoulders in and during this process.

When you spend a long time feeling lonely and isolated, it can feel like you're carrying around so many insecurities and secrets. But, once I decided it was time to deal with these issues, I quicky realised how incredibly liberating and therapeutic facing up to your problems can be. I've now a new outlook on life and have never felt better about myself. When I look back at my life, I often think my teens, twenties and thirties could be considered as a write off. I now feel I'm finally living the life I want to live.

My Condition, My Life

You often remember certain comments or phrases from your childhood that stick in your head. For me it was being told I was a 'big kid.' I wasn't overweight, I was just tall for my age. When you're reminded of comments from people saying, 'he's too big to be in a pram. Or he's too big to be playing with those toys'. These comments stick in your head. It may sound inconsequential to many but, for me, that phrase followed me around like an old penny. A penny I did not want in my pocket.

When I think back to my childhood, I remember being relatively content. I played sports, I had friends, went to birthday parties etc. However, what did have an impact on me was changing schools at the age of nine. This happened because we moved house and out to the countryside of county Dublin. I was taken away from my friends. I felt very isolated and lonely at our new home. We had money and on the outside, everything appeared rosy, I became very introverted and lost all confidence in myself. There weren't many kids around to make friends with, but I did make some. To this day, some of them are still my best friends but they never knew the turmoil that was happening in my head.

At thirteen, I was enrolled in lifesaving classes at our local swimming club. Our family friends' daughters had attended these, so they recommended myself and my sister also try out the classes. With my self-esteem already incredibly low, this was not the environment I needed at the time. The boys had to wear bathing trunks (Speedos) we were not allowed wear shorts. Looking back now, I felt very exposed and self-conscious. We would have to stand at the side of the pool in front of everyone and rehearse lifesaving scenarios. My heart would be beating out of my chest, my anxiety would be through the roof and I just wanted to run to the changing rooms and seek sanctuary. I would be dreading going to these classes all week. When the class would finish, I couldn't wait to get home and go straight to my bedroom and burst into tears. I attended those classes for most of my teens, and at the age of eighteen I finished attending. But the damage was done. I was broken.

I sought help and attended therapy in my early 20s for depression. I remember one of the first questions the therapist asked me was, how am I feeling? The analogy I used to describe my existence was like a 'walking corpse'. I felt empty inside and would cry a lot, constantly have negative thoughts about myself and would want to end my life. I disliked my chin, my ears, my hair, my wrists, my waist, everything. I even hated me looking at my own shadow. My continual dislike for myself would control everything. And it continued into my thirties. By that time, the rot had set in. When you tell yourself you hate everything about yourself every day, you eventually believe it. I had stopped going out, seeing my friends, going to the gym etc. I would look away if someone pulled up beside me in traffic as I didn't like my side profile in their car windows.

I hated seeing my reflection. It was mentally and physically draining keeping up this façade.

Therapy helped ease the depression, but the negative thoughts about myself continued.

I attended therapy in my thirties as I was changing careers and my mental health just wasn't strong enough to cope with the demands of retraining and entering a new workplace environment. I was diagnosed with Generalised Anxiety Disorder. Both times I attended therapy, but I never once mentioned my issues with my body image or my binge eating. I guess I wasn't ready to discuss these topics. I admitted them in private to myself, but not to anyone else. I was self-stigmatising myself. Men don't have body image issues, right? Men don't have food issues either?

My thirties, just like my twenties and my teens, were a write off in my own head. I didn't want to think or talk about them. I was happy to stay in the shadows and sweep everything under the rug. But, that was all about to change.

Hope For Me & Millennials

The themes for this year's volume of Mental Health For Millennials are Inclusion and Hope. These are two topics close to my heart. Over the years, I've felt excluded from society, friends and family. All my own doing I might add. I've felt there was no hope for me. However, I've come a long way in the past year. Twelve months ago I was sitting at home, pondering my thoughts as the pandemic was well and truly upon us. I didn't feel anxious about staying home, so many people I spoke to who live with anxiety were basically feeling a sense of comfort with not having to leave the house. Their social anxiety was being put to one side for the time being.

As I sat at my home work station, I was as usual, questioning everything and allowing my thoughts to 'spiral'. Several people had previously suggested that I try journaling because it can be very cathartic and also help transfer your thoughts from your head to a page or screen. I was sceptical, I guess I just didn't want to deal with the possibility of floodgates opening in my life and overwhelming me with feelings and emotions I wasn't used to dealing with. Also, I'm a guy; why would I write down my thoughts? How can that be beneficial?

The blog evolved into a blogging site and podcast called 'The Endless Spiral'. It was a name that came quickly to me for obvious reasons. I had wanted to share some aspects of my story for a while, but I guess I felt the timing wasn't right.

With The Endless Spiral, I wanted to provide people with a platform to share their stories via blogs, vlogs, or by joining me on the podcast for a chat. I was incredibly inspired by the amazing guests who contributed to the podcast and blog. I began to write more blogs myself and speak more openly about my own story. The floodgates were slowly beginning to open and flood my life with thoughts, memories and emotions which I had buried a long time ago.

I was soon introduced to the terms, <u>Body Dysmorphia</u> Disorder and <u>Binge Eating Disorder</u> and my life changed overnight. I now had a label for how I had been feeling for over twenty years. It was a huge weight lifted off my shoulders. After a few Google searches, a light bulb went on above my head. If these feelings and actions have names, perhaps there is a solution. My story quickly shifted from using sport as an escapism (I used that word rather than saying I was in denial) to raising awareness for BDD and BED. Sharing my story provided me with a plethora of resources, connections and information.

I've learned so much about myself and about the conditions I've been living with for so long, and it feels incredible. I've never felt better about myself than I do right now. I've learned to trust my body to tell me when I'm hungry and when I'm full. I've learned to exercise to affect how I feel rather than how I look. I've learned to use gratitude. I now do yoga and practice mindfulness.

I used to believe that if I looked better on the outside, I would feel better on the inside. This is fine for some people, but I had issues that went deeper. Everything I did was for the wrong reasons. I was focusing on the neck down and forgetting about the neck up. I would starve myself and then binge. I'd then want to purge, and the spiral would begin again. I would feel anxious at the gym. I wouldn't go out, I stepped into the shadows and there. I stayed for a long time.

Once I established a healthy relationship with myself, I was able to establish a healthy relationship with everything else. It may appear simple, but I would never have discovered this if I had kept everything bottled up.

Take Away Nuggets

- Some have said, that I've been through more in twelve months than others have in five years. It's not a race; go at your own pace; you'll get there eventually. But you must take the first step.
- If I could speak to my younger self what would I say? I'll close with some words of wisdom: no matter your age, gender, shape, or size, everyone can struggle with food and body image.
- Keep in mind that it's never too late to seek help. This is something I can attest to. I'm now in my early forties and I feel like I'm starting life all over again. Don't hide, there's no shame in asking for help, share your experiences, and talk to someone.

I can assure you that you are not alone.

- I now process feelings, emotions and situations differently. This didn't happen overnight; it's taken hard work and a lot of self-development. When I look back at my younger self, I sometimes ask myself, would I do anything differently? I guess, one thing I would say to myself is, don't live inside your own head. When you live inside your head you only have your own perspective to listen to, and that's more often than not, negative. Don't be afraid to share, you'd be surprised how many people close to you will be supportive.

- Aside from giving myself some words of advice, I wouldn't actually change anything. I wouldn't be the person I am today if I hadn't gone through some difficult situations.

Are Recent Movements Towards an Inclusive Model in Irish Education Promoting the Caring Side of Education?

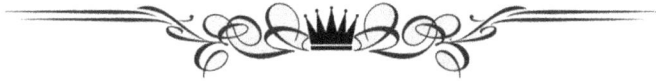

Anne Marie Doyle, M.Ed.

Introduction

Irish millennials have lived through a significant fast-paced journey while the Irish Education System has moved towards providing an inclusive education for those with Special Educational Needs (SEN), with much progression happening over the last twenty years. Older millennials may currently have children traversing an education system which is quite different to the one they experienced growing up and younger millennials attended school just as some of the most progressive steps toward inclusion took place. As an older millennial, a primary school teacher of twenty years, a deputy principal of over ten years and currently working as a special education teacher, I have seen these changes first hand, and learned as much as I could about inclusion by doing further studies in psychology, autism and inclusive education.

In terms of the Irish Education System, the goal of inclusion sets out to build a framework within which differences between individuals are accepted, accommodated and championed. Inclusion doesn't seek to erase or ignore these differences. Indeed, inclusion implies the right to what is understood to be an appropriate education (Department of Education and Science, 2007).

With this in mind, we look to see how Ireland has moved towards creating inclusive education. It was in 1993 that the Department of Education underlined some of the shortfalls in the education system in terms of meeting the needs of all children in mainstream primary classrooms. Many children with additional needs were being taught by way of segregation via institutions or separate teaching environments (Department of Education and Science, 1993). In 2001, a Task Report Review outlined that teachers and personnel working with students with additional needs should have an in-depth knowledge of disorders and of the most current methodologies being used to achieve educational and social success for students with diverse needs. (Department of Education and Science, 2001). The EPSEN Act (2004) envisaged that people with additional needs would be enabled to participate in an inclusive society and to live independent lives following an education which supported their individual needs and strengths.

Following on from these policy changes and recommendations during the last twenty years in particular, fewer children are enrolling in special schools and more children with additional needs are attending their local mainstream primary school (Banks and McCoy, 2017). An investment in staff resources, such as providing increased special education teaching hours and allocating Special Needs Assistants (SNAs) to those with communication, behaviour and care needs, made attending a local mainstream primary school accessible. Children who would have been unable to attend school without extra adult assistance have increasingly been given the support needed to scaffold their learning towards independence – this has been a great source of hope for the future in terms of facilitating the sense of belonging for all adults in an inclusive society. Many schools are still over relying on withdrawing students from their classroom to be educated separately from their peers during the school day (Rose, Shevlin, Winer & O'Raw, 2015). Of course, this is absolutely necessary in teaching specific skills, but giving more support in-class has generally been advised to meet learners needs in an inclusive manner, so that students interact and are educated with their peers, leading to a greater sense of self-esteem and a sense of school belonging (Department of Education and Science, 2017).

Studies have found that the presence of Special Needs Assistants (SNAs) has enhanced the student experience, with learners appreciating the helpful support of these workers, who assist students to stay on task and to progress towards independence as they advance through the classes alongside their peers in their school (Rose et al, 2015). Other studies have also found that SNAs have helped to foster independence while they support and care for students. Many students feel that SNAs support their mental health, as SNAs have often been described as a friend who helped them to manage their behaviour, to calm down and to de-escalate situations that were overstimulating (Griffin, 2018). In fact, SNA assistance has been described as therapeutic and a boost to well-being (Logan, 2008) as SNAs help give students a sense of belonging and community and facilitate them to have meaningful participation in their classroom. Increasingly, school staff have been given more training to help manage behaviour, which requires an elevated level of expertise, so that school staff have the responding, reactive and preventative skills necessary to protect students if they are finding it difficult to self-soothe when upset. This may help teachers to manage and react to their students better, but it also puts a lot of pressure on school staff. A protocol in reacting to volatile behaviour is essential in de-escalating the risk for children themselves and for bystanders. Understanding the complexities of behaviour and the reasons for emotional and behavioural difficulties that children experience has increasingly been established as an expertise that is necessary for managing challenging behaviour (Zhao et al, 2021) and indeed for providing a nurturing, caring environment for learners. This investment in terms of upskilling teachers and SNAs, is certainly a cause for optimism in terms of a commitment to fostering the success of all students in nurturing mainstream, inclusive settings. Establishing belonging, promoting achievement and delivering appropriate education provision for all has resulted in a rise in the number of children with additional needs attending mainstream primary schools due to the national policy and legislation changes, particularly in the last two decades.

The changes that have occurred during the years when our younger millennials were attending school and our older millennials have begun to have children traversing the school system gives us hope that our society has become a more caring, inclusive society in the last twenty years. Children with diverse needs are increasingly being taught alongside their neighbours and peers from their community rather than being separated or indeed segregated from children their own age who live near them. This, in turn, has no doubt helped their peers to gain a better understanding of children with additional needs that they may not have met or encountered in the past. The need for parents to drive past their local school gate, which must have been heart-breaking for many, is not happening to the same extent as it was in the past.

In my own experience, and during research that I did as part of my Master of Education (Special and Inclusive Education), I have found that developing social skills is seen as a very important factor as we prepare learners for experiencing independence and success in society. Developing friendship skills both in the classroom and in the yard, helps children to feel a sense of belonging and community. Teachers and SNAs have a caring role in the community, whereby they help to enhance the well-being, self-esteem and overall mental health of students. When children are going through a tough time emotionally, they can access nurturing, therapeutic programmes alongside sensory activities and rooms in their schools.

Unfortunately, during my research I realised that overcrowded Irish classrooms were not always the environment that was best suited to supporting the emotional needs and well-being of all children with many school staff reporting that we have class sizes of over 30, above the European average. School classrooms are often buzzing hives of activity, and for many this is a positive experience, but some children find this kind of noise overwhelming and overstimulating. They need quieter, calmer environments. While this is increasingly being facilitated with SNA and Special Education Teacher (SET) support, there is often not enough space or personnel available to provide the optimum level of care and assistance. Furthermore, while upskilling is happening, it is often self-funded by school personnel as they endeavour to provide the best support to the children in their care. There are often waiting lists for teachers to access essential professional development that they need in order to provide an inclusive environment for all, this seems to be a finance issue, with not enough courses being made available due to funding.

Nonetheless, there is certainly a great feeling of hope for our developing inclusive society, that cares about all citizens and puts a stop to segregation as many of our millennials begin to enrol their children in school. Some of the obstacles that still exist can be removed easily. There is certainly a feeling of hope, as we see how many steps have been taken during the lives of millennials to create a more caring, inclusive society. We have achieved so much in a short space of time and there is certainly a feeling that mainstream schools are trying to promote the best interests and the overall well-being of their students, while they nurture their sense of belonging and well-being and respond to the diverse needs of children with a greater knowledge than before.

Takeaway Points for Millennials

- Policy changes in the last 20 years have meant that more children with additional needs are enrolling in mainstream primary schools than in special schools.
- Special Education Teachers and Special Needs Assistants are encouraged to have expertise in the area of special needs so that they can support the success, well-being and mental health of students.
- Children with additional needs are increasingly being taught inside their classroom, rather than being withdrawn for extra support in another room, to facilitate peer interactions, a sense of belonging and community and overall well-being. There is a classroom support plan in place to scaffold them towards success.

- All school personnel are encouraged to upskill so that optimum support can be provided for students with diverse needs to help them to develop independence as we strive to create a more inclusive society.
- Barriers are being removed as awareness develops. Our society is becoming more understanding as educators, and all citizens, learn more about the diverse needs of others. This sense of care facilitates inclusion and helps us to look after the mental-health of others.

> *"Do the best you can until you know better.*
> *Then, when you know better, do better."*
>
> —Maya Angelou

References

Banks, J., Frawley, D., & McCoy, S. (2015). Achieving Inclusion: Effective resourcing of students with special educational needs. *International Journal of Inclusive Education*, 19, pp 926-943.

Department of Education and Science. (1993). Report of the Special Education Review Committee (SERC), Dublin.

Department of Education and Science. (2001). Educational Provision and Support for Persons with Autistic Spectrum Disorders: The Report of the Task Force on Autism. Dublin.

Department of Education and Science. (2007). Inclusion of Students with Special Educational Needs Post-Primary Guidelines. Dublin.

Department of Education and Skills. (2017). Guidelines for Primary Schools Supporting Pupils with Special Educational Needs in Mainstream Schools. Dublin

EPSEN Act. (2004) *The Education for Persons with Special Educational Needs Act.* Dublin: Department of Education and Science/The Stationery Office.

Griffin, C. (2018). Fostering Independence through Care? A Study of the Preparedness and Deployment of Special Needs Assistants When Supporting Pupils' Behavioural Care Needs and Independence Development in Mainstream Primary Schools in Ireland. Unpublished doctoral dissertation. Institute of Education, University College London.

Logan, A. 2008. Special needs and children's rights to be heard under the UN Convention of the Rights of the Child 1989 in the Republic of Ireland. *Education Law Journal*, 9(2), pp 1–14.

Rose, R., Shevlin, M., Winter, E., & O'Raw, P. (2015). Project IRIS–Inclusive research in Irish schools. A Longitudinal Study of the Experiences of and Outcomes for Pupils with Special Educational Needs (SEN) in Irish Schools. NCSE: Meath

Zhao, Y., Richard, R., & Shevlin, M. (2021). Paraprofessional Support in Irish Schools: From Special Needs Assistants to Inclusion Support Assistants. *European Journal of Special Needs Education* 36(2) pp 183-97.

My Soundtrack to Hope

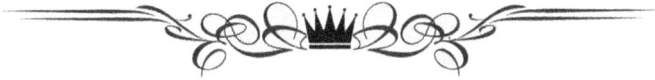

Chris Sherlock, Broadcaster

*H*ope. It's a word I believe we use just as much as, "Hello…how are you?" It's all around us, whether it's hoping you get that new job you wanted, hope to love again after a break-up, or the hope to pass a driving test. For me, it was the hope to enjoy life again by coming out of my self-imposed isolation, otherwise known as "my comfort zone." I've spoken before about my personal story of how I was victimised through a series of brutal bullying tactics by classmates in *Mental Health for Millennials* (volume 4; 2020). And though it took time, patience and consistent effort, it was music that offered me the hope that better days were yet to be.

The bullying prevented me from safely returning to secondary school. I was rather sadly left to my own devices when budget cuts took away home tuition. Without the funding for the tutors needed to pass my exams, I was in a kind of limbo. It felt like education-purgatory. Besides trying to continue my studies on my own, I was also dealing with more personal problems because of the psychological damage caused by bullying. Anxiety, depression and stress all came crashing down around me. When I had to leave my house for appointments, shopping, walks or even to go to group events (especially when I didn't know anyone at these events), I would look for the nearest exits and be ready to leave as quick as my legs could take me in the fear of experiencing more bullying.

There were times when hope was barely a glimmer during those dark days. But there were good days, too—a lot more good than bad thankfully! In that rollercoaster time period, I discovered my true passion and decided to pursue a career in broadcasting. A job where I knew I'd be in the public eye, opening me up to potential ridicule, and yes, the possibility of future bullying. There was so much to absorb about the business. I did all I could to research media outlets like radio, but the biggest lesson learned in making the career choice I made was that it was okay to trust others again.

Would I get made fun of? Would someone else try to hurt me? Most students moving on from secondary school don't have to worry about those things, whether moving on to university or entering the work force. I did though. Bullying held me back...but not for long. After about two years, I found the courage to engage more with people. Before that, my social circle was small--just friends and family who'd already earned my trust. Counselling helped. I had to learn to not only trust others again, but to trust myself as well. My confidence and self-esteem needed a big boost, and part of that came with remembering that I was actually a people-person who was outgoing, funny and even an occasional prankster. It's remarkable how much of yourself you lose when you've experienced bullying—that aspect is often ignored. But it's why I'm not only writing this chapter, but also why I've become an anti-bullying campaigner since I first published my story. The thought of someone else going through what I did is almost as painful as the initial experience.

Wanting to incorporate that sense of self (along with my quirky sense of humour) into my career somehow along with my love of music was a natural fit for radio. Being a radio presenter seemed the perfect way for me to dip my toe in the broadcasting waters, and I've never looked back since. My love for music was my saving grace; it was always playing in the house when I was a growing up. One minute, you could hear Helen Shapiro's "Walking Back to Happiness," then maybe something by Michael Jackson or Cliff Richard—perhaps even a 90's dance tune that would (sometimes literally) rattle the fillings in your teeth.

Music brings with it so much diversity. There is nothing like hearing a great ballad, but it's just as wonderful to listen to a simple sing-along tune or even one you can just hum and sway along with. Sadly, I can't sing or write music but have family involved in the business and now know many more artists whom I'm proud to call my friends. Seeing the release of a new tune gets me excited and I enjoy being supportive of the talented musicians of all varieties. Some let me into their world and though I'm no Simon Cowell, it's always a great compliment when my feedback is valued as if I were.

I'm lucky enough to listen to some of the best Irish music available and include as many Irish artists as possible on my radio shows. Some of those gifted musicians are unsigned and just trying to get their music out to anyone willing to listen. Giving artists that kind of hope is part of what I love most about my job today. My career in broadcasting is everything I wished for and more. I really enjoy meeting new people, playing music, chatting about plays/movies/books—even being subject to a brain hack thanks to Irish magician and mentalist, Keith Barry. These are things I would have missed out on if I didn't have the hope, courage and determination to continue on with my life goals after being bullied.

Chris Sherlock

I remember first seeing the Flirt FM volunteer poster on the grounds of National University of Ireland in Galway—it was my chance to give broadcasting a try and follow my path. Today, I feel like I was born to do radio and work with musicians. Hope is what got me here. Having the ability to talk the arse off a kettle and squeeze in some music! It's great, the journey has begun and I'm enjoying every second.

Music has been the soundtrack of hope to my life. But these songs I'm sharing here are ones that keep me inspired to push on with my dreams. There's a song I came to know over the years, "Isle Of Hope, Isle of Tears" written by Brendan Graham (1997) and performed by Mary Duff; it's been covered by many Irish artists, including Sean Keane, Celtic Thunder, and Celtic Woman, to name but a few. Celtic Woman's version is my favourite; the song tells the story of the first Irish immigrant to enter America through Ellis Island in 1892, 15 year old Annie Moore. The song goes on to talk about how Annie was leaving everything behind and starting over in a new place. It compares Ireland - the isle of tears - and the Isle of Manhattan – the isle of hope.

Annie's story is relatable to anyone who wants to make a better life for themselves; she did that by taking the road less travelled. Annie needed the hope that she could have her own happily ever after. Ireland was facing dark times in 1892. Poverty was prevalent. There wasn't much hope for young people like Annie. While my story may seem completely different on the surface, I, too, took a big risk, like Annie. My dark times included the trauma of being bullied during a formative period of my life. Music gave me the hope to set sail on my own journey toward freedom—a journey that has led me to go from an introverted, shy nervous teenager to the outgoing and outspoken man I've become.

My current sense of hope is connected to my desire to continue working within the Radio & TV broadcasting community. Though inclusion is all about diversity and is absolutely needed in our society, as a white male, it's incredible to reflect on how bullying disenfranchised me to the point where I did not feel like I was a part of larger society. One can only imagine the level of difficulty for people who are not part of heteronormative ideals. It's my wish for the world that all people of every race, ethnicity, culture and religious background can find hope to move forward. It's important to include diverse individuals in every area of society. After the bullying isolated me from my peers, it's a relief to feel so accepted within the field of broadcasting. From the minute I walked in the Flirt FM studios, I felt at home. Today, that sense of acceptance has allowed me to open up with my personal bullying story in not just this book series, *Mental Health for Millennials*, but on local and national radio, newspapers and podcasts as an anti-bullying campaigner.

Going public with my story wasn't easy—it brought up the real fear of re-traumatisation. But when in doubt, breathe! I took my own advice and remembered that the sky wasn't going to come crashing down. It was a great help that all the presenters, researchers, producers and journalists I've worked with on the anti-bullying campaign trail have been so friendly. Their kindness and care coming with compassion, not judgement—this only increased my sense that I was working in the right field. It's exciting to know deep down that the media world is where I belong. Being included in the workplace is a must; it doesn't matter the job you're in, we all aim to make sure we put food on the table and pay our bills with the hope to have fun along the way. Going on holidays to visit family and friends abroad, taking in a concert, making sure the kids are provided for…everyone has high hopes for what their careers can do for them, and why not? We all deserve a fair and equal chance to not only survive but to thrive. Hope lives in that space.

"High Hopes" is a song that rocketed up the charts, written and performed by Panic at the Disco (2018). The overall theme and message of the song is that no matter how hard your dreams seem, just keep going! As you may tell by now, I really listen to the lyrics in music and enjoy the riffs, melodies, etc., all of which I have learned thanks to working in the entertainment industry. When dealing with mental health battles, my hobbies saved me. Spending time focusing on my strengths brought me back to myself. I listened to medical professionals, yes, but I also took note of what was around me and while rest is always needed to heal, putting energy into your ambitions and goals can build confidence and self-esteem while also creating a sense of fun and laughter.

P.T. Barnum said these great sayings "Comfort is the enemy of progress," and "Your success depends on what you do yourself, with your own means."[4] In case you don't know who this guy is, he was an American showman and is known for creating the circus. Until P. T. Barnum dreamt of the circus, it did not exist. People around Barnum thought he was insane. Who would go to a circus??? Everyone. Everyone wanted to go and everyone went. Barnum's "crazy" idea was suddenly the norm. In many ways, the idea of a kid who could not complete his schooling thanks to bullies to becoming a broadcaster may seem equally unlikely to naysayers. But like Barnum, I have both hope and faith in myself and my dreams. I am going to continue working toward my goals,

---

[4] "Though I reference Barnum as an entertainment visionary, he was also a fallible human being noted in history for exploiting people of colour, in particular Joice Heth and Aboriginal people from Australia. In no way, shape or form do I condone Barnum's actions. My introduction to him was through the American film, *The Greatest Showman* (2017), starring Hugh Jackman; Barnum was portrayed as a musically-inclined and very relatable underdog in the film and did not reflect the true history of Barnum or the origins of his circus."

no matter what. And if that gives others hope to do the same, then sharing my story is worth the effort.

Challenges keep one motivated. Motivation helps us to consistently move toward our goals. I believe it's good to always take on a personal challenge whenever you can, no matter how big or small. That's part of hope…having the faith that we can move forward, even in the face of seemingly insurmountable odds. Speaking of which, I mentioned that I can't sing, dance, act, nor play any instruments, yet I'm still working in the entertainment industry. If you want something badly enough, nothing can stop you. Part of what helped me break into a field I had no training or talents in was that I was unafraid to turn to those who have what I lack. I may never be a famous singer, songwriter, or musician, but I can support them. That's how I found my niche.

Songs that I have on my playlist to this day are inspired by hope and happiness. Whitney Houston and Mariah Carey sing, "When You Believe" (1998) written by Jewish composer, Stephen Schwartz—it's about the story of Passover, a Jewish holiday. Moses is sent by God to deliver the Jewish people from slavery in Egypt, but he doesn't have the confidence to do it. Even though he grew up with the Pharoah as his brother, Moses felt insecure. We can see a fictionalised version of this biblical tale play out in *The Prince of Egypt*, the animated movie that the Houston-Carey song was written for. The overall message is that when you believe in miracles, they will happen. It's about positive psychology, first developed by an American Jewish professor named Martin Seligman. There's no small coincidence there, as the Jewish people have dealt with anti-Semitism that swept Europe during World War II, and regrettably, even manifested in Ireland. To listen to a song encouraging people to believe in miracles that comes from a community who has been targeted by bullies for millennia is beyond hopeful. The idea that an entire nation can come back and stand tall after millions were murdered in the Holocaust also reminds me of "Hopeful" performed by Bars & Melody, a 2014 song about anti-bullying and being hopeful enough to experience a new day. The Jewish people have certainly done that and managed to inspire many more around the world to do the same— including me.

I'd like to close by sharing more music, this from the Irish group, The Coronas: "Write Our Own Soundtrack" (2021) is based on how a new relationship can give you hope and positivity when the world is falling apart. "High Hopes" written and performed by Kodaline which is based on positive psychology and may help those reading this to find hope in dark times. Finally, I've got to mention, "Don't Give Up," written and performed by Nathan Grisdale (2019); it is a song that was sent into me at the radio station and is among many of my favourites. The lyrics and meaning are so simple yet so meaningful. The title is self-explanatory with its uplifting message and I would like to encourage you to take a real listen to these songs.

If you appreciate music like I do, then why not make your own hope and inspirational soundtrack??? It will always be there when you need it: YOUR CHOICE. YOUR FAVOURITES. YOUR WAY!

Inclusiveness and Hope in Education: Millennial Master's Life During a Global Pandemic

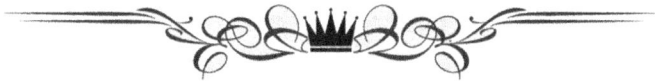

Sinéad O'Malley

Introduction

The rapid onset of the COVID-19 pandemic in 2020 caused major disruption and volatility across the globe, including in the education system in Ireland. The education system needed to find a means of continuing the delivery of education since it was unclear whether face-to-face lecturing would be able to continue due to health concerns. As a result of on-campus learning coming to a complete halt, online learning was deemed a suitable temporary remedy to the issue (Singh *et al.* 2020). However, McGrath *et al.* (2021) argue that the series of changes the pandemic has brought with regard to education have, in fact, been a long time coming. As education was disrupted so significantly, it was forced to adapt quickly and create suitable changes which, without the outbreak of

Covid, may have taken many years to introduce (Ó Caollaí, 2021).

When I began my nervous and uncertain pursuit of returning to 3ʳᵈ level education during the first lockdown in 2020, the idea of hope was certainly a factor in my decision making. I was faced with leaving a comfortable and happy full-time job in pursuit of something that had been on my mind for a number of years – a Master's degree. During a time when spirits were undoubtedly at their lowest and many felt lost, including myself, I was inspired to take on that new challenge in my life. Upon reflection, I now feel this may not have been possible if it wasn't for the pandemic and the changes it brought to everyone's lives.

Millennial Mental Health during the Pandemic

According to Deloitte's Millennial Survey (2021) approximately one third of respondents reported having taken time off from their jobs due to feelings of anxiety and stress during Covid. Of those respondents who did not take time off work, four in ten classified themselves as 'stressed all of the time' however they chose to push through these feelings and continue working. An overall conclusion from this survey highlighted a stark reality that as a direct result of the onset of Covid 19, both Millennials and Gen Zs are significantly more pessimistic of worldviews and are experiencing major levels of anxiety in comparison to any other time that they have been evaluated for this survey.

On a daily basis, Millennials are making use of numerous different technological devices and systems in order to sustain relationships with their family and peers (Weda *et al.* 2022). In another study conducted on Millennials by Mockaitis and Butler (2020) it was found that among participants surveyed, a paradox exists between the notion that Millennials, who are often associated with being technology savvy, did actually have the most difficult time coping with the rippling effects of the pandemic. Generational change is not by any means a new concept as every generation is exposed to various global events, advancements in technology and social norms, which all heavily influence the way in which people respond and shape what is most important to individuals in that particular generation (Hopkins *et al.* 2018).

> *'As a whole, millennials have been described as well-educated, optimistic, collaborative, sociable, and open-minded'*
>
> (Raines, 2003).

Blended Learning

The concept of blended learning is not an entirely new method of learning as it has been used for approximately the last two decades and there have been numerous definitions and changes to the overall concept (Alammary *et al.* 2014). Blended learning is described as 'learning activities that involve a systematic combination of co-present or face-to-face interactions and technologically mediated interactions between students, teachers and learning resources' (Bliuc *et al.* 2007, p.234).

Benefits of a blended learning approach to 3rd level education are numerous. They include enhanced autonomy for learning, increased opportunities for students, mutual cost effectiveness and greater geographical and time flexibility for both students and lecturers (Smith and Hill, 2018). The Organisation for Economic Co-operation and Development (OECD) supports this view, whereby the development of digital technologies holds immense potential to drastically improve both the quality of delivery and equity in third level education and, if implemented correctly, could increase access to non-traditional learners, lower educational expenses, and enhance customised and adaptable learning (OECD, 2021). As the population in higher and adult education becomes increasingly diversified, the requirement for connecting remote individual students has grown exponentially. For example, 'Lifelong learners' are frequently unable to attend regular classroom training for a myriad of reasons which can include family or employment obligations (Raes *et al.* 2020).

However, like many things, I wish to acknowledge some potential disadvantages of a blended learning approach. These include time management, the plethora of issues associated with the use of technology, decreased integration between students and lecturers and a possibility of an increased workload (Anthony, 2021).

Nevertheless, as a millennial, I would like to see a continuous mixture of both face-to-face learning and remote learning. This is because, I feel by encouraging this it is a more inclusive way of teaching and casts a wider net to all people aspiring to add to their educational achievements. This, of course, is only my opinion. However, having experienced third level education in both pre and post pandemic settings, I can see the difference it can make to people's lives.

In September 2020, I began a postgrad in Business at NUI Galway. I chose this course because it seemed to be the perfect transition course to getting me where I wanted to be having studied Social Care in my undergrad degree. The course itself was to be held in person, however, Covid has put a stop to that. Though the course was held online for the entirety of the semester, there was always a glimmer of hope that we, as a class, would make it to campus and all meet face-to-face. This was not meant to be unfortunately. Upon reflection, the frantic efforts of my group members and myself trying to put reports and presentations together for assignments over Teams and Zoom despite having never met each other is, in my opinion, testament to the resilient and adaptable nature of millennials themselves.

I was fortunate enough when I began my Masters in Human Resource Management in September 2021, when relatively normal on-campus activities started to resume. I cannot express how grateful I am for the opportunity to meet my fellow classmates on the first day of the Masters in Human Resource Management and feel that that opportunity was lost in the postgrad the previous year. Along with the mixture of nerves, I felt immense feelings of hope at the beginning of that semester. And a lot of this stems from the ability to meet new friends with similar mindsets, interests and goals.

Keeping in line with the theme of this volume, the idea of inclusivity was paramount here. The difference in the ability to mix with friends and be face-to-face with lecturers was instrumental in my learning, overall feelings of inclusion and my whole university experience. A sense of belonging is also, in my opinion, crucial to university success.

As a millennial, I can directly relate to Gabrielova and Buchko (2021) when they describe how millennials flourish from work that challenges them and are appreciative of any feedback from authoritative figures coupled with a strong desire for organisational participation and support.

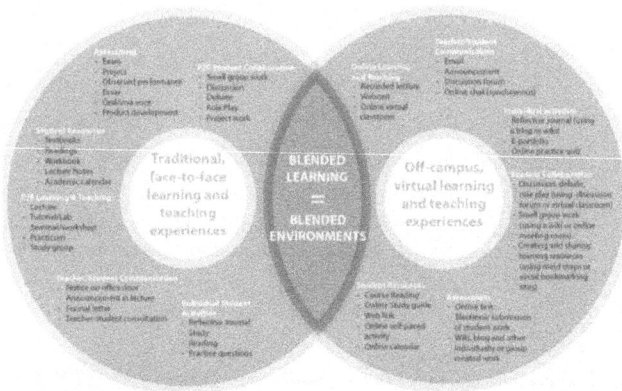

Source: Griffith University (2010): Getting started with Blended Learning

In essence, I can appreciate both sides of the coin here. There are many pros and cons to both on-campus face-to-face learning and remote learning. I believe, based on my own experience, that third level institutions should implement a blended learning model which would take into account and include all students' lifestyles, abilities and scope for learning. Having spent two whole years in full-time postgraduate education during the pandemic, I feel grateful most of all for the support and encouragement from my parents and family.

'A lack of belonging will increase the risk of alienation, burnout and underperformance'
—(Chamorro-Premuzic and Berg, 2021).

Learning Nuggets:

- I would encourage anyone who is thinking about upskilling in any way, to go for it. It is not an easy route, but the outcome far outweighs the hardship.
- Taking on a challenge like a course, or learning a new skill, is so important when it comes to self-development.

Be the person
that
Makes
others feel
Included

References

Alammary, A., Sheard, J., Carbone, A. (2014). Blended learning in higher education: Three different design approaches. *Australasian Journal of Educational Technology,* 30(4) 440-454. DOI: https://doi.org/10.14742/ajet.693

Anthony, B. (2021). An exploratory study on academic staff perception towards blended learning in higher education. *Education and Information Technologies,* https://doi.org/10.1007/s10639-021-10705-x

Bliuc, A.M., Goodyear, P., & Ellis, R.A. (2007). Research focus and methodological choices in studies into students' experiences of blended learning in higher education. *Internet and Higher Education,* 10(4) 231-244. https://doi.org/10.1016/j.iheduc.2007.08.001

Deloitte (2021) The Deloitte Global 2021 Millennial and Gen Z Survey. https://www2.deloitte.com/content/dam/Deloitte/global/Documents/2021-deloitte-global-millennial-survey-report.pdf

Chamorro-Premuzic, T., & Berg, K. (2021). Fostering a Culture of Belonging in the Hybrid Workplace. *Harvard Business Review,* https://hbr.org/2021/08/fostering-a-culture-of-belonging-in-the-hybrid-workplace

Gabrielova, K., & Buchko, A. (2021). Here comes Generation Z: Millennials as managers. *Business Horizons,* 64(4) 489-499. https://doi.org/10.1016/j.bushor.2021.02.013

Griffith University (2010). Getting started with Blended Learning. https://www.griffith.ie/admissions/blended-online/what-blended-learning

Hopkins, L., Hampton, B. S., Abbott, J. F., Buery-Joyner, S.D., Craig, L.B., Dalrymple, J., Ramsey, S.M. (2018). To the point: medical education, technology, and the millennial learner. *American Journal of Obstetrics and Gynecology,* 218(2), 188-192. https://www.sciencedirect.com/journal/american-journal-of-obstetrics-and-gynecology/vol/218/issue/2

McGrath, C., Palmgren, P., & Liljedahl, M. (2021). Beyond brick and mortar: Staying connected in post-pandemic blended learning environments. *Medical Education,* 55(8) 890-891. https://doi.org/10.1111/medu.14546

Mockaitis, A., Butler, C. (2020). Disrupted: Remote Work and Life under Lockdown during the Great COVID-19 Pause. https://mockaitisdotcom.files.wordpress.com/2020/07/report-july-2020-study-1.docx-1.pdf

Ó Caollaí, E., (2021). Online and upwards: Preparing for autumn return to third-level. *The Irish Times,* June 1, https://www.irishtimes.com/news/education/online-and-upwards-preparing-for-autumn-return-to-third-level-1.4574999

OECD (2021). Higher Education Policy. https://www.oecd.org/education/higher-education-policy/

Raes, A., Loulou., D. Windey, I., & Depaepe., F. (2020). A systematic literature review on synchronous hybrid learning: gaps identified. *Learning Environments Research,* 3(3) 269-290. https://link.springer.com/article/10.1007/s10984-019-09303-z

Raines, C., (2003). Connecting generations: The sourcebook for a new workplace. Thomson Crisp Learning.

Singh, J., Evans, E., Reed, A., Karch, L., Qualey, K., Singh, L., & Wiersma, H. (2020). Online, Hybrid, and Face to-Face Learning Through the Eyes of Faculty, Students, Administrators, and Instructional Designers: Lessons Learned and Directions for the Post-Vaccine and Post-Pandemic/COVID-19 World. *Journal of Educational Technology Systems,* 50(3) 301–326. https://journals.sagepub.com/doi/10.1177/00472395211063754

Smith, K., & Hill, J., (2018). Defining the nature of blended learning through its depiction in current research. *Higher Education Research & Development,* 38(2) 383-397. https://doi-org.nuigalway.idm.oclc.org/10.1080/07294360.2018.1517732

Weda, S., Rahman, F., Samad, I., Gunawan, F., & Fitriani, S., (2022). How Millennials Can Promote Social Harmony through Intercultural Communication at Higher Education. *Randwick International of Social Sciences,* 3(1) 231-243. DOI: https://doi.org/10.47175/rissj.v3i1.398

A New Hope...Episode VI:
An Garda Siochana, Millennials and a Culture of
Hope and Inclusion

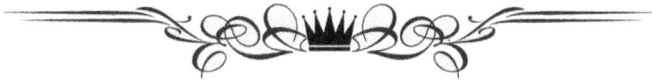

Ray Flannery

Now, I know the eagle eyed observers and, more importantly, the Star Wars aficionados among you may have noticed the faux pas in the title of my chapter, but I can guarantee you that it is intended. Star Wars fans... I apologise. For once, the much maligned millennial is the receiver of praise from this particular author, and not the subject of my angst.

Those of you who know me, will now that I have been a proud member of An Garda Siochana for the past thirty one years. I can still fondly recall my first day walking into a Garda station in the big bad capital and absolutely bricking it. I looked around me at these giants of men and women and sat in awe of them, whilst listening to their war stories of "the good auld days". The way they spoke in admiration of these fabled no nonsense individuals, who policed Dublin in a certain manner, a manner which I may add would not be tolerated in today's society, simply amazed this raw recruit from the country.

I can still remember thinking to myself that things were different now and that I was going to be one of the new members to "make a difference" but in a far more modern and sophisticated way.

Following on from The Walsh Report (1985) on Garda Probationer Training, things changed. I was one of this new breed of Garda, unlike the old system of six month training in Templemore, our training was for a two year period overall. This would consist of college time, work experience, more college and then a probationary period of being let loose on the streets. There was a huge expectation of hope in the upper echelons of the force that, because of this new method of training, we were going to be better equipped to meet the latest in the line of hardened criminals on the streets. We were the first recruits to be afforded the opportunity to see the different areas the job had to offer ranging from drugs, forensics, serious crime, terrorism etc. For us, this was an amazing opportunity to gain experience in the different fields that the job had to offer. We got little taster placements with these high profile units which, in turn, pushed us to concentrate on the necessary requirements needed in order to nail down a permanent position with these elite units. Of course, this engendered a sense of resentment in some of the aforementioned elder lemons. How dare these young pups simply step over them into these positions, we hadn't served our time in their eyes.

Of course, there was the usual smart arse comments from the elder lemons towards us young pups who thought that we knew it all after a few weeks on the job. After all, the majority of new recruits had not just joined up straight from school, no, in fact we had those among us with college degrees or work experience from other areas in life. We had a different outlook to life in comparison to many of the older members. WE WERE DIFFERENT! We asked the questions that the more senior member wouldn't ask. Strangely though, all our newly acquired wisdom didn't count for much in the real world of dealing with criminals. Now, I am not saying that there were no benefits from the new training, because there most certainly was. For starters, we did tend to use our brains quicker than our brawn. We saw people in a different light to our predecessors and treated them accordingly. We did have the advantage of being psychologically educated and also having the wherewithal to use this training wherever possible.

Over the years, I have witnessed the attitudes of a variety of colleagues toward criminality, ethnicity, promotion, and in just basically dealing with the public. When I joined, you were told to know your place when it came to promotion, to know when to offer an opinion and more importantly when not to offer one. This is where the millennial comes into his/her own. In the first instance, the millennial now expects diversity and demands equality. This is a cultural mind shift. The millennial also will expect to work with people from all areas of life, of all genders, religions, races. Up to this year, promotion in the force consisted of studying for an exam, if successful, two interviews and if you happened to have someone of a higher rank fighting your corner or fell into the nepotism category, you stood a good chance of going up the ranks. Today however, that is gone. Now it's a psychometric test, followed by an interview and that is it. The old "pull" is gone. The best person should now be getting the promotion. The millennial thinks that this is how it always should have been. I totally agree and I for one, am delighted to see such progression. Little room for cronyism these days!

As a result of having been in the force for almost all of my working life, I am not qualified and, therefore, not in a position to write critically about millennials in the private sector. Save for the very many conversations I have had with friends who do operate in the "real world" as I am often reminded of their status. I do, however, read articles that pique my interest and I am aware of a recent survey carried out by Deloitte University (2014; 2015) into millennials which I found fascinating. I am fully aware that the millennial is purpose driven in their work; they are very capable and competent of inventing alternative ways of getting things done. Unlike in my profession where change is slow and new work practises can be frowned upon by the dinosaurs of old.

Yes, before you say it, I am fully cognisant of the fact that I am now one of the dinosaurs. I am all for methods, devices etc that will enable the work to be more streamlined and practical. Off the top of my head, I can think of twenty things which would improve the efficiency of the job and its methods. The millennial does not buy into the theory of "this is how the job was always done". They see an opportunity to change things and they grasp this with both hands. In my opinion, the only downside of this as far as I can see is that the mentality of the Gardai being a 'job for life' is gone. As a result of this, the loyalty factor is missing and, indeed, this is a common thread in human resources (Murphy, 2022).

During my career, I have a few friends I have acquired through the years, I have had loads of acquaintances, colleagues, but few whom I would trust my innermost secrets to. In work, I would trust them with my life and the brotherhood and sisterhood within the job when things unfortunately go wrong. They had my back. The millennial, however, appears more content to resign and head for pastures new. This, in a strange way, gives me hope. Millennials don't care what others will say if they leave employment and move elsewhere. If it is not for them, or they see a better opportunity elsewhere, then its 'adios'. The monthly inhouse bulletin showing promotions, moves, retirements and resignations has made for very interesting reading over the last few years.

Another area in which I have seen major change has been in the recruitment of nationals who have come from different backgrounds, countries and race. This has to be of huge benefit to the force. The ability to be able to call on the different experiences and qualifications that these people have to offer is simply something money can't buy. The force as a rule had been stuck in a time warp but thanks to a modern way of thinking which I fully believe has been brought about by the many millennials entering the job, there is loads of change on the horizon. I never thought I would see a uniform garda sporting a beard or turban, I also never thought I would see a new practical uniform being worn by members but today both are in evidence.

The millennial doesn't see the obstacles within the job previously witnessed by people like myself and if they do encounter these obstacles, they simply adapt and overcome (as much as the job will allow!) We haven't always been the most forward thinking outfit after all. The fact that the millennial sees the diversity of race, philosophies, thoughts, as 'normal' has led to them utilising this to their advantage. Every opinion is valued and every voice is heard. The millennial also believes, according to the Deloitte survey, that current leadership and the cultures within organisations are too traditional and inward looking. The 2014 study also pointed out that the millennial is fully aware that they do not have the same depth of experience that we old-timers do but, they see this as a huge opportunity to redefine a leader's role and even more importantly, they have the tools and the confidence to put this into practice. This, of course, brings human resource challenges.

The millennial also is far more conscious of having a good work-life balance and, as is the title of this series of books, are far more conscious of the advantages of not only physical but mental health. Back in my early career if I had had the misfortune to deal with a traumatic incident, be it an accident, murder, fire etc, it was usually followed by a trip to a public house and the downing of copious amounts of alcohol to help get your mind off things. If a visit to a counsellor was even mentioned, it would be laughed off in an instant by some of my peers. I find it so encouraging to see the younger members, millennials being so open about seeking help if and when it is needed. From my own personal experience, I have had some of these conversations with these members. They have come looking for advice in some instances and in others, merely to have a chat. I am all too aware that they see me as one of the senior members, even though we would share the same rank. It is amazing what can be revealed over a cup of coffee. I will offer advice if I am in a position to offer same, if not, I will point them in the right direction to someone who has expertise in the area. The days of bottling things up are hopefully in the past and this is a giant step forward for millennials in policing.

So, in conclusion, I am a happy camper. I see a bright future for An Garda Síochána and society in general. The days of being told what to and how to do it from a group of people ill qualified to offer such advice, are coming to an end. Millennials are a breath of fresh air to An Garda Síochána. I don't say this lightly either. They refuse to be shackled to the old methods. They have an intelligence and are not one bit afraid of utilising this intelligence and have the balls to offer an opinion or disagree with one if they can see a different solution to the problem at hand. If the millennials were to adopt the military motto of "To adapt and overcome" it might be a stretch but only a tiny one in my humble opinion.

The millennial generation has demanded and stood up for change and have achieved this change at least to a degree that brings hope. Their wish to be included and be inclusive is refreshing. This is what brings me such hope on both a personal and professional level. As I stated earlier, the millennial expects diversity and inclusion, and rightly so. Ireland has led the way in recent years in changing the way society thinks and acts, the smoking ban, plastic bag levies, gay marriage etc, and for this I think this little island of ours deserves a pat on the back.

References

The Deloitte University Leadership Centre for Inclusion.

Deloitte (2014) Millennial Survey

Deloitte (2015) Millennial Survey

Gallup poll 2015

Boston College Centre for Work and Family Research (2015)

The Garda Training Committee Report on Probationer Training 1985 (Walsh Report)

'Be A Man' in the Modern World

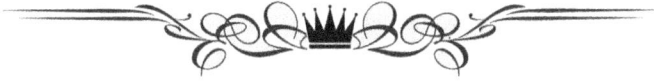

Daragh Fleming

At time of writing I am 27 years old. Which means I am a millennial. I am a man. I am also a man who talks about his emotions and mental health. Which is rare. But not as rare as it once was. There was a time in that not so distance past where even the idea of being vulnerable was simply not something a man could consider. Only 10 years ago I lost my best friend to suicide and had no idea he was struggling. In the 10 years since Erbie died, we've gone from mental health not really being talked about at all to mental health being addressed nearly everywhere, and that is incredibly uplifting. I believe that if Erbie was alive today, he may not have died by suicide because he may feel like it would okay for him to express himself. So in this sense we're in a very hopeful and exciting moment for men's mental health, but we still have some ways to go.

I'm sure you know by now that men account for three quarters of all suicides. That's quite staggering, and this statistic speaks to the problems men face with their mental health. Men are brought up as children to chin up, to be strong, and to generally be stoic. None of these things are bad on their own, but when you are repeatedly told that this is the way you should be then you begin to believe that behaving in any other way is wrong.

This is the problem more so than anything – it's not that men are told they should be strong, it's that we believe that we cannot be vulnerable.

Men struggle to open up about their emotions. I have in the past. I know that at times I've struggled and kept it to myself because I've felt ashamed. I've had panic attacks in the safety of my room and never told a soul about them. Men find it difficult to open up because they feel like they're supposed to be strong and get over things without ever really addressing them. Men feel like they can't open up because society has taught us in many different ways that this is simply not what men do.

It's understandable, really. If you spend your whole childhood and adolescence being scorned and mocked by your peers for showing any sign of emotion it's only natural that you'll do anything you can to learn how to bottle these emotions up. Being teased for crying or feeling sad, or whatever it may be, was so commonplace growing up. Any lads in my school who more effeminate than other boys were the butt of most jokes. If that is your default, and your norm of existence, I'm sure you would learn to stop sharing how you feel too. Adults often tell boys to stop crying when they're upset. 'Be a man' has often been synonymous with being unemotional. But there is no law of physics or of the universe that has ever stated that men cannot feel emotions. What a truly ridiculous concept that is.

Being a man in today's world can be challenging because, although you are encouraged now more than ever to talk, it simultaneously feels like this world sometimes despises men. I've often seen men open up about how they're feeling only to be told that how they are feeling about a situation is wrong. If all feelings are valid, and men should talk about how they feel, how on Earth can they be wrong to feel the way they feel? It sometimes seems like people are happy to hear you speak about your emotions, so long what you say is convenient.

What would you do in a situation where you know you want to talk about how you feel, because you've been told it's okay, but you also fear the backlash for saying how you feel? Would you risk opening up or would you continue to struggle in silence like you always have? Today's world is more encouraging for men than ever before but there's still far more men dying by suicide than any other group, and so there has to be something else going on. Perhaps being encouraged isn't enough. Perhaps being told to be more like women, and to resist our masculinity isn't the answer. Men and women are different biologically. That's a fact. And so too are there social, physical, and psychological differences. Our needs are not the same, and so a one-size-fits-all solution for mental health may not be what's required. Perhaps the reason men struggle with their mental health is because they are told to deal with their struggles in the same ways women do. Perhaps this is ineffective, and maybe we need coping mechanisms specific to the needs of men.

I can comfortably open up about how I'm feeling now, but I couldn't always do that. And for a long time, I've been the outlier in my group of friends, talking openly and casually when I'm feeling anxious or sad, or frustrated. I've been to all-boys schools and been on sports teams. Men and boys don't generally just say how they're feeling. Instead they mask it with jokes, or refer to how they're feeling nonchalantly as if it's no big deal. The men I've observed throughout my life will rarely sit down with a cup of tea and talk about their feelings, but I've heard countless revelations and releases during training sessions, on runs and in the gym. Of course, some men do sit down and talk it out. What I'm saying is there is more than one way to go about it, and there are no wrong answers in this sense. There is no 'right' way to express your emotions, and so maybe men just need different avenues in order to express themselves.

And addressing the men's mental health crisis won't just benefit the men who are struggling but will actually benefit all of society. For it is men who are unable to properly address their trauma or deal with their emotions who often become dangerous, violent and oppressive. And so, in many ways addressing the men's mental health crisis seriously throughout society we can hopefully mitigate many instances of male violence.

As such, it is pivotal that issues affecting men are directly addressed in order to stop these terrible atrocities perpetrated by some dangerous men.

Change takes time. In a very short amount of time, we've gone from men being expected to stay strong and silent, to men being encouraged to talk about their emotions. This is very good undoubtedly, but it's not something that will take root everywhere overnight. Men are still scarred by their upbringings. Men are still afraid of the backlash that might come with saying the wrong thing. But we'll get there, and hopefully when we do, less men will feel like they have to take their own lives. Less men will feel isolated and lonely and they'll tell their friends how they feel and get the help they deserve.

Some Advice

Ignore the voice telling you that you should not feel the way you are feeling. We all have this voice. It's the voice which also tells you that you should not cry, or that you just need to get over yourself. This voice lies to us, and as men, I think we listen to it far too often.

I think the best thing men can do for themselves is understand that we do have emotions and we are entitled to feel them. It doesn't make you any less of a man to feel your feelings. It baffles me that we got to a point where society expects men to be non-feeling and unaffected all the time. It's neither realistic nor helpful.

I promise you that you will feel so much better if you talk to even one person about how you feel. It doesn't even have to be this colossal conversation. It can be casual and comfortable. Pick one person you trust and have a conversation about how you've been feeling. Really and genuinely reflect on what has made you anxious, or sad, or frustrated this week and let it all out. You don't need to tell the world, but you do need to tell someone.

I'm a man who's previously been caught in the belief that I am not 'allowed' to struggle, and that it is un-manly to have emotions. Now I'm still a man, but I no longer believe these things, and I'm better for it.

Across your lifespan you will hear other men, and even women, say awful things about men who are open and vulnerable and comfortable with their emotions. It comes with the territory. My advice to you is to not only ignore these voices, but to understand that these sentiments are coming from people who are also struggling and hurting, who have problems of their own which they may not be dealing with. They may be taking out their frustrations on you, as a man, because it's a low hanging fruit. If we can understand that this is what is going on, we can rise above it and move on.

Just because someone says something about you, doesn't make it true – in fact in most cases it's the furthest thing from true.

The take home is here is that you are a human being before you are a man, and human beings feel emotions. You are allowed to feel the way you feel, and you are certainly allowed to talk about it too.

A Hopeful Conclusion

Society impacts us all in unequal ways because society in imperfect. And the reason it is imperfect is because it comes about via imperfect beings – ourselves. Rather than looking at our issues through a divisive lens we should look at things from a place of togetherness to improve areas that need improving. On social media today, many of us get caught up in identity politics and begin to miss what is truly important. We care more about being right, or having our opinions heard than we do about the causes we shout about, and many people who need the most help are left to fall through the cracks.

Men's mental health is but one of these issues, but it is often one that is neglected due to a modern attitude of disdain towards men in general. Divisiveness such as this only adds to the problems at hand rather than helping to improve things. We must resist allowing our emotions and egos to dictate how we respond to such issues. We must acknowledge that blaming entire demographics for the acts of individuals is objectively immoral in all contexts. If we can do these things then I believe we'll be able to address all of our societal issues effectively, including the male mental health crisis.

And that certainly fills me with hope.

Take Away Nuggets

- Being a man doesn't mean you don't have emotions, nor does it mean that you should not have them. Being a man means being able to express yourself in healthy ways, by addressing your emotional reality and adapting.

- I don't think there is anything objectively wrong with masculinity. The modern world often suggests the opposite. But being masculine doesn't make you 'bad'. Rather it was what you do as an individual person which defines you.

- Talking about your mental health will not fix your problems entirely, but it will certainly help you to feel better in the moment. Trust me on that one.

- Find out what works for your mental health. We're all different, and so what works for me may not necessarily work for you. There is no blanket approach that will suit all people, or all genders. Spend time finding methods that work for you and develop a mental health routine.

- Above all else – look for the good in this world. It's certainly there. Our modern world tends to focus on the negative at times and this can work to drag us down with it. Focusing on what is good in your life, no matter how benign, is a damned better way to be than to become bitter and resentful. I think that's the difference between a life with hope and a life without it.

Reference

Platt, S. (2017). Suicide in men: what is the problem? *Trends in Urology & Men's Health*, 8(4), 9-12.

Holding Onto Positivity Everyday

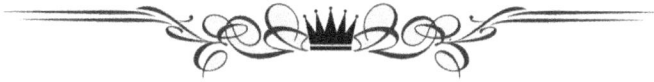

Karen Gallen

ope is an inspiring word, but it is often used flippantly – 'I hope you have a good day' or 'I hope you enjoy your lunch' etc. But, to me it is an aspiration and alludes to endless possibilities. As a parent to a beautiful teenager with additional needs, every day I live with hope – some days I hope for a (positive) diagnosis, other days I hope for a miracle and other times still, I hope for better days. Presently, all hope is pinned on what is proposed by her surgeon to be her final spinal surgery (spinal fusion) which is scheduled to take place in April this year. An end to eleven years of trips to theatre and the hope that with a fused and somewhat straighter spine, she will take the final step in her surgical adventures and an unaided physical step in the real world.

This journey of hers commenced in the second year of her life and in November 2021 the gauntlet was thrown down. The

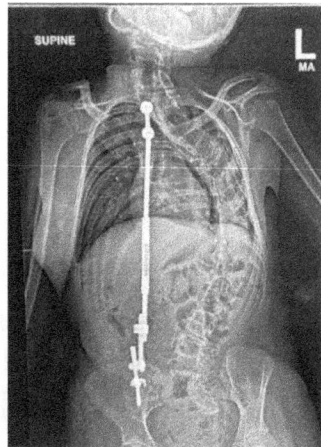

words I wanted to hear yet dreaded hearing, were spoken in a busy Day Ward at Temple Street Children's Hospital in Dublin, Ireland. As I reflect, I feel as though I heard them under water... muffled but comprehensible "Next step for your daughter is fusion." In that instant, the surgery she was about to have that day went out of focus and significance and my head was catapulted into the future. But I know we must live in the present.

Fast forward to February 2022 and I gaze down at my porch floor where the post has landed...Face up with the familiar addressee 'Parents/Guardians of Saoirse Gallen' and the bright red post mark of the hospital in the top right-hand corner. Reality check!!!! Before I opened the letter, I knew it was her pre-op assessment date and nervous excitement caused me to call my closest confidants to make the announcement that 'this is really happening'.

So, the date given for the pre op assessment was 18th February, 2022 and all I could think of was that 'I can weather this storm.' And a storm it was. The day before the appointment, weather warnings were issued by Met Eireann and Storm Eunice crossed the country meaning an overnight in Dublin to avoid hazardous weather conditions and to ensure that it was possible to attend the hospital. At 9.00am Saoirse and I entered the Day Ward for literally a day long assessment. We took our place at her appointed bed and waited in both fear and trepidation for the endless flow of therapists to visit and impart their information and expertise and also answer my endless questions. The day started with a consultation with two physiotherapists, followed by the spinal nurse, then an occupational therapist, then an echo and ECG performed by the cardiologist, followed by the dietitian, then phlebotomy and finally the anaesthetics team. A mountain of information whirling around in my head, the scariest being that she would be approximately seven hours in theatre with her spinal cord being monitored constantly while she is operated on, that she will go to ICU immediately post-surgery, will be on a ventilator and have a nasal feeding tube for a number of days.

To be honest, I was glad to have been given the opportunity to prepare for what will happen as being forewarned means you are forearmed but I also was glad to have all of these experts in addition to the Professor in Orthopaedics and his surgical team on our side. The journey home was filled with an air of expectancy and hope. And the waiting game begins…

An initial verbal date was given for April 2022 and then changed to May 2022 so when no letter arrived giving a specific theatre date, I contacted the Spinal Nurse. It was agreed that 10th June, 2022 would be 'the big day' subject to an ICU bed being available. So, between 19th May, 2022 and 9th June, 2022 I asked the universe to make it happen and to keep Covid from our house. The universe obliged – thankfully.

Prior to the surgery date, a lot of organising and arranging had to be done. The one issue being accommodation for me during her hospital stay. There are a number of rooms available onsite in the hospital in Parent's Accommodation however they are demand led so I joined the waiting list. In the interim, I tried to book a hotel in close proximity to the hospital and what I like to call 'the additional invisible stresses' began to unfold. My stomach churned when I received a quotation for 8 nights in a single room with no breakfast which amounted to almost €2,200. In a state of disbelief and anger, I posted about the exorbitant costs on Twitter and much to my amazement, I received an unbelievable outpouring of support and also numerous and extremely generous of offers of accommodation in houses in Dublin, plus use of cars, offers of lifts to hospital. Most offers were received through Twitter and some through other social media platforms from people who had read my post on Twitter with over 276,000 engagements with my post.

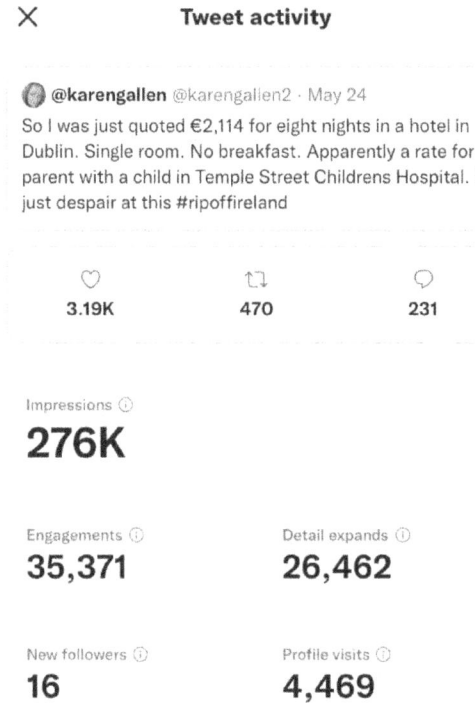

✕   **Tweet activity**

@karengallen @karengallen2 · May 24

So I was just quoted €2,114 for eight nights in a hotel in Dublin. Single room. No breakfast. Apparently a rate for a parent with a child in Temple Street Childrens Hospital. I just despair at this #ripoffireland

♡   ⟲   ♡
3.19K   470   231

Impressions ⓘ
276K

Engagements ⓘ   Detail expands ⓘ
35,371   **26,462**

New followers ⓘ   Profile visits ⓘ
16   **4,469**

People really are amazing at their core, and I will be forever grateful to those who offered assistance both publicly and privately. I am pleased to say that I ended up staying in Hugh's House which is a charity that offers accommodation to families who have children in Temple Street Hospital, Holles Street, The Coombe and The Rotunda 365 days a year.

On the day prior to theatre, we were admitted to St. Michael's B Ward and that day and night seemed endless as no ICU bed was available at 7pm that evening. I hoped and hoped all night that the situation would change and that a child would be discharged from ICU as the anaesthetics team said that surgery would not proceed without a guaranteed ICU bed. Finally, at 6.45am on the Friday morning, a nurse popped her head around the curtains of the bed and left a theatre gown – the relief was immense but also short lived because although it is what I wanted to happen, I was extremely anxious deep down inside.

At 7.45am we were escorted to the theatre floor and after numerous checks etc, we began the long walk to the operating room. It is such a brightly lit area that it is startling to the senses. No number of visits will ever dim this perception for me. I placed my daughter on the operating table and sat on a stool beside her, holding her hand, desperately trying not to look around me. However, curiosity killed the cat, so I glanced around fleetingly and the room seemed full of people and equipment – more so than other visits so I focused completely on squeezing my daughter's hand and saying repeatedly 'I'm here'. A mask with anaesthetic gases was placed over her mouth and her eyes started to close and suddenly I heard the words I dislike so much 'now mum, she's asleep now and you can go. We'll look after her and she'll be back to you shortly'. *Short* is not a word I'd use to describe time when you can't control the situation and when you're separated from your child. I left theatre, put my gown and cap in the bin and fled down the backstairs crying. Some things never change…

At 10am, I sat on her bed in the ward holding her toy dog and I saw her surgeon approach me. I leapt to my feet, immediately asking what was wrong. He came to discuss options for surgery. Now, anyone who has been to theatre is aware this is discussed well in advance, however the options and approach he was supposed to follow were now not viable. We discussed an alternative approach and I am thankful that he included me as part of that decision making process. My reply to him was to bring her back safe to me and that I trusted him implicitly.

Several hours later, I was buzzed into ICU and I am not sure if my heart flipped or my stomach somersaulted. She had the appearance of a small, porcelain doll, overshadowed by wires and machines. I felt sick. I still feel sick when I think about this. She had multiple IV lines, a central line, drain from her back etc Everything seemed surreal. Isolated in a room with a nurse by her side, constantly checking and rechecking her stats. I felt overwhelmed and also awkward because this was beyond my experience of over thirty theatre visits. I am pleased to say that she only spent a day and a half there before being relocated to Surgical Flat. The remaining days were a blur and I had to check my phone to see what day it was regularly. A never-ending cycle of medicines, checking her stats and trying to reposition her. One day, the physio exercise was to higher up the head rest on her bed, the next day was for her to sit at the edge of the bed whilst being supported from the front and behind, then it was to stand, then take some steps. There was a lot of 'ouch' and 'I'm sore' being used but gentle persuasion, bribery and pleading saw us through those days and eventually we got the go ahead to travel home by Bumbleance. Bumbleance is an ambulance service which is designed for newborn babies to 18 year-olds and is the official Children's National Ambulance Service of Ireland. Richard, our driver, made the journey home as smooth and as comfortable as possible.

Time has passed since we came home on 17th June and recovery is slow, but it is still recovery. Children are so resilient and full of hope. Every day I am asked by her as to when we are going to the farm, on holidays, to school (especially school). Of course, at the time of writing this at the start of week two in July she is only sitting out for short periods and taking five-minute walks, but the hope and enthusiasm are there.

It has been an eventful journey to get to this point in her life and so many lessons have been learned:

1. Never give up hope. Despite waiting for surgery, it did happen eventually and was successful.
2. Those that care stick with you through the bad times.
3. Accept any help given, from the grandest gesture to a silly meme or a call from someone who cares.
4. Support comes in many forms; from people you know in real life to online support groups.
5. It's never too late to upskill (as I have learned). I can now strip a bed and change the bed covers with a person still lying in it (courtesy of onsite training from the staff in the hospital).
6. I now know that I turn to humour to deflect what is happening during difficult times.

Onwards and upwardly mobile is how I see my daughter's future. Perseverance and hope have brought her to where she is today. These may not be the answer to every life question/problem but it does help.

'Never lose hope, my dear heart, miracles dwell in the invisible.'

—Rumi

The Ever-Burning Flame Of Hope Experienced By Those Working in Irish Agriculture

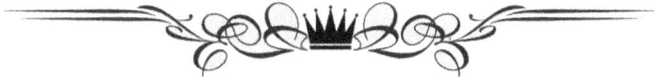

Anne Hayden

"Nothing should be out of the reach of hope. Life is a hope".
—Oscar Wilde, 1893 (A Woman of No Importance)

Introduction

This chapter will explore hope in an Irish agricultural context, how it affects the psyche of farmers, along with the importance of establishing a successor and, in particular, the women who work in agriculture both as farmers and in support roles. This essay is written from my personal point of view as a millennial woman working in Irish agriculture and my hope for the future of women in this industry. I am from the 9ᵗʰ generation of an Irish farming family, and I am currently undertaking my PhD in agricultural economics and so agriculture, women's role and the hope that is ever-present in this profession is a topic that I am deeply passionate about and fascinated by.

Hope is a universal theme that is experienced in every facet of Irish life but none so much as in Irish agriculture. In an agricultural context, hope comes in two forms; firstly, that of hope for the role and place of farms in Irish agriculture and its continued place of importance in society; and secondly, the hope for Irish women who are entering into and are carving out new roles in Irish agriculture.

I will discuss how hope has been defined and interpreted and the unique and intrinsic role that hope plays amongst both Irish farmers and in broader agriculture. I will examine the rising optimism that is currently experienced by Irish women working in agriculture as they actively redefine their role in this sector.

The Requirement and Ever Presence of Hope in Irish Agriculture

Hope, while not discussed on a regular basis in mainstream agricultural publications, is a crucial driving factor as to why farmers choose to enter into and stay in the farming profession. Hope, simplistically put, is defined as a desire that sits alongside an expectation of obtaining what is desired or a belief that it is, somehow, obtainable (Magaletta and Oliver, 1999). It is this desire and expectation that is ingrained into the psyche of young farmers that contribute to their propensity to return and work their land even when it is not economically viable or, indeed, profitable to do so. The idea of hope is a key stone of Irish agriculture as farmers continue to plant crops for the next harvest even if this years has not been particularly successful or profitable in the hope that the next year will be better.

However, this idea of hope among farmers does not merely go as far as just the production of agricultural goods, but it also helps to provide farmers with a deep-rooted attachment to the land with the inherent hope that future generations will continue in their endeavours. The concept of being attached to the farmland and it not being solely for the production of agricultural goods illustrate this broader concept of social belonging by connecting these farmers with and within the wider community in which they operate.

The experiences and the links farmers feel to the land and their rural communities, as well as their homeplace, determine whether they wish to return to live and work there in the future (Cassidy, 2010). People's sense of cultural identity, as well as their own personal identity, is intertwined with their identity of place and, in part, the idea of the loss of this sense of place; there are more dimensions to this than just a physical place that includes emotional, symbolic and cultural dimensions (Buttimer and Seamon, 2015). These factors stem from the underlying current of optimism and hope that these young farmers experience which plays a vital role in the establishment of a successor for the agricultural enterprise. Without this hope, a successor would not be willing to take on the enterprise, and this would have catastrophic results for farming.

The relationship between agricultural succession and economic viability can thus be characterised as circular and interdependent (Duesberg et al., 2017). This relationship is also complex but can be simplified as the economic viability of certain farming types having an effect on the willingness of a successor to be established; however, without investment in new technologies, these farms are likely to be less profitable, but it is more likely that only younger farmers will make these necessary investments (Calus et al., 2008; Donnellan, 2019).

In rural Ireland today there are more older farmers than younger farmers, despite it being proven in research and practice that young farmers have a positive impact on a farm's economic viability as well as adopting more environmentally friendly farming practices. According to the Farm Structural Data in Ireland in 2016, there were 137,500 farms in Ireland, but of these, 7,800 farmers were operated by farmers under the age of thirty-five, while 41,200 farms were operated by farmers over the age of sixty-five (CSO, 2019). Traditionally, the attitudes and values toward farming in Ireland centred around the presence of a male heir as a successor as an integral factor in the decision to continue the family farm.

The Evolving Role of Women in Irish Agriculture

At present, in Ireland, the workforce of Irish women in farming is only 13% which puts women in the minority; however, to quote Bob Dylan, "the times are a-changing," and in particular, this was supported in the latest Common Agricultural Policy reform proposal. This proposed reform included an increased rate of grant aid of 60% for women over the age of 40 under the Targeted Agriculture Modernisation Schemes (TAMS) and with the included option of attending women-only knowledge transfer groups. Previously less than 4% of TAMS grants were awarded to female farmers. As part of this proposed CAP reform, it is estimated by The Women in Agriculture Stakeholder Group chair Hanna Quinn Mulligan that this will change the lives of 70,000 women working across farms in Ireland who have been described by many working in the industry on social media and anecdotally as previously being effectively voiceless and invisible up to now, which is a remarkable milestone towards equality in Irish agriculture.

This movement and change in attitudes toward women and the role that they play in Irish agriculture have been echoed by the Irish government, and as a millennial woman working in this sector, it fills me with hope to see the past contributions as well as the current contributions that women have made to the agricultural sector finally being given the recognition that they deserve.

This movement has been slow and long overdue, to say the least, and while officially in Ireland, there are only 16,000 registered women farmers, it is estimated by the Central Statistics Office for Ireland (CSO) that every day 70,000 women are farming yet go unrecognised for their actions. I, like many women working in the agricultural field, gain great encouragement from the changes that we see developing before us, not only at a national level and with the positive changes to support that has been seen recently, but also socially where there has been a shift in the attitudes towards women entering into agriculture. According to the Irish farm relief services, there has been a steady increase in women opting to study agriculture in college (Marks, 2019). Along with this, anecdotally, there has also been an increase in the use of social media such as Instagram and TikTok by young female farmers to increase awareness of their role and occupation. I have found these posts so inspiring that I might even commence posting myself! These posts provide support and a community for women who are entering into and are at present farming.

Conclusion

As I reflect on the continuous development of Irish agriculture and perhaps the most important lesson that I have learnt in my 28 years as part of a farming family, it is the ever-persistent idea of hope and optimism. With the economic variability that is associated with working in agriculture, hope is a persistent and necessary outlook to have if one is to continue to work in this field.

My choice to enter into the agricultural profession was widely met with approval from my family and dearest friends, but other millennial women have not been met with the same support. In fact, recently, women in agriculture on Instagram and other social media platforms have been sharing both their positive and negative experiences some of the particularly antiquated attitudes that they have to endure daily working in agriculture. However, I am hopeful that these attitudes are changing and will soon become a thing of the past. As Oscar Wilde said so eloquently, "nothing should be out of the reach of hope", and I am confident with continued support, the number of younger farmers and, in particular, the number of young female farmers in Ireland will continue to grow. Eventually, my hope for the sector is that gender equality is achieved and that the barriers to working in agriculture will be less of an issue but till that day, I continue to remain hopeful not only for the survival of the agricultural industry in Ireland but that it will thrive for future generations to come.

As I have seen first-hand among the millennials working in Irish agriculture hope must be constantly cultivated as otherwise it will impossible to enter into or stay in the profession. While agriculture is an extremely rewarding profession, it is predominantly a solo enterprise and it can be an isolating profession, so it is very important that we check in with our mental health and to make time to see friends and family as well as connect with people who are going through similar experiences. Through the likes of these support groups such as Teagasc and women in agriculture they can offer support and advice to people going through similar situations. These lessons and reminders to look after our mental health, find support and ask for help it when we need it, as well as cultivating hope in our profession are not limited to just us working in the agriculture profession but are universal and should be embraced by all of us in our chosen professions and day to day life.

References

Buttimer, A., Seamon, D., 2015. The Human Experience of Space and Place. Routledge.

Calus, M., Huylenbroeck, G.V., Lierde, D.V., 2008. The Relationship between Farm Succession and Farm Assets on Belgian Farms. Sociol. Rural. 48, 38–56. https://doi.org/10.1111/j.1467-9523.2008.00448.x

Cassidy, A., 2010. 'I'm not going to be able to leave': The impact of belonging to the Irish farming community on university students' life experiences and transitions to adulthood. 405.

CSO, 2019. Statistical Yearbook of Ireland 2018 [WWW Document]. URL https://www.cso.ie/en/releasesandpublications/ep/p-syi/psyi2018/agri/farmsandfarmers/ (accessed 3.31.22).

DAFM, 2021. Minister McConalogue announces supports to promote gender equality in farming [WWW Document]. URL https://www.gov.ie/ga/preasraitis/c9232-minister-mcconalogue-announces-supports-to-promote-gender-equality-in-farming/ (accessed 3.31.22).

Donnellan, T., 2019. Ireland: The likely effects of full decoupling.

Duesberg, S., Bogue, P., Renwick, A., 2017. Retirement farming or sustainable growth – land transfer choices for farmers without a successor. Land Use Policy 61, 526–535. https://doi.org/10.1016/j.landusepol.2016.12.007

Magaletta, P.R., Oliver, J.M., 1999. The hope construct, will, and ways: Their relations with self-efficacy, optimism, and general well-being. J. Clin. Psychol. 55, 539–551. https://doi.org/10.1002/(SICI)1097-4679(199905)55:5<539::AID-JCLP2>3.0.CO;2-G

Marks, J., 2019. Increase in the number of students, particularly women studying agriculture [WWW Document]. FRS Farm Relief Serv. URL https://frsfarmreliefservices.ie/article-an-increase-in-the-number-of-students-particularly-women-opting-to-study-agriculture/ (accessed 3.31.22).

The Long Journey Home

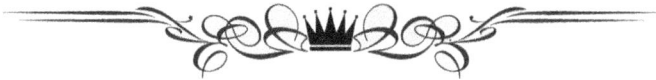

Jantien Schoenmakers

O n May 29th 2018, a Tuesday, I was supposed to fly home to the Netherlands with my (then) almost 3 year old son. Due to thunderstorms at Schiphol Airport, our flight from Dublin got delayed and then cancelled. Aer Lingus put us in a nice hotel near the airport for the night and booked us on a flight home in the morning. My son and I safely got the flight the following day, but when I arrived at Schiphol Airport and went to the bathroom before the car ride home, I noticed I was bleeding. At 18 weeks pregnant, I knew that was a bad sign and asked my mother to drive me to the hospital where my old rheumatologist was, as I knew they would still have my medical details on file.

On arrival at Accident & Emergency, the triage nurse asked me how many weeks along I was? They rang the department and, after a few minutes, two nurses came down with a wheelchair for me. The nurses still managed to crack a joke or two whilst trying to comfort me. When I arrived upstairs, the doctor did an ultrasound and after a few minutes my worst nightmare came true: there was no heartbeat from the foetus.

The doctor asked the consultant for a second opinion to be sure, but still no heartbeat.

My beautiful baby had passed away.

A plan of action was discussed with the obstetrician for the following days. There was no rush to deliver the baby as there were no signs of infection. They were going to induce labour on the Saturday, giving my partner time to fly over so he could be there during delivery. I rang the bookshop where he worked from the hospital. After he told his manager what happened, she instructed him to use the work computer to book a plane ticket and head home to pack his bag straight away. I was told to go home to my mother's house and rest up, and that they would see me back in Amsterdam on Saturday morning.

Instead of going to her house, my mother, my son and I went to her mobile home in the countryside, so he could have some more freedom, go swimming and play outside. My hope was to, at least, make it feel like a holiday for him, even if I didn't feel like that at all. When we got there, we sat ourselves down on the deck outside. Two of my mother's friends came by and congratulated me on my pregnancy. They meant well but it actually broke me. All the grief came over me like a tsunami and I went inside to have a good cry and have a few minutes to myself. My mother told them what had happened and made sure the news spread so no more people would come by and do the same thing.

The next day we drove back up to Amsterdam and picked up my partner from the airport. For someone who is extremely private about everything, I couldn't keep it together and cried in his arms when he came out of the terminal. I had never been more relieved to see anyone as he was my rock. He made sure that I knew he was going to be there for support, but also that we were going to get through this. That everything was going to be alright. Even if it was going to be the most difficult and painful thing we had ever done as a couple.

Friday June 1st. Dinner in the little restaurant, the Pavillion, on the campsite. A medium-rare steak with extra garlic butter, as I didn't have to mind what foods I was eating anymore. The cramps started. I thought it was the amount of food I had eaten, but quickly realised they were contractions. I asked my mother to drive us to the hospital in Amsterdam. She asked whether or not I wanted to go to the hospital in Rotterdam or Amsterdam as the latter had my records, it was the hospital I had attended on Wednesday and they were expecting me the following day. Amsterdam was the obvious choice. On the way there, 'You'll Be in My Heart' by Phil Collins came on the radio. I cried, and realised this was the song that was forever going to be related to my stillborn baby.

When I arrived at the hospital, the gynaecology department nurses were expecting me and the two that came down with a wheelchair were the same two nurses who wheeled me up on Wednesday. When they helped me into the bed, I realised this and said one was the same nurse who was funny in the hallways on Wednesday, to which she replied that she was also funny in other places. They told my partner he could stay with me all night and that they would get him a fold out bed later.

The medical side of things kicked in. The nurse checked how far I was dilated, and asked if I wanted pain medication for the contractions and labour. She checked my bloods as I had been diagnosed with Systemic Lupus Erythematosus a decade before and she wanted to make sure my blood levels were all okay. She gave me an injection of morphine and I gave birth to a beautiful baby boy, who had passed on but genuinely looked like he was sleeping peacefully. At 18 weeks, he was absolutely tiny and could fit in the palm of my hand. They asked if I wanted to cut the umbilical cord, which I did. My placenta wasn't coming out by itself, and I had to be put under full anaesthetic for a retained placenta D&C to remove it.

When I came back from recovery, the nurses had looked after my partner and set up the fold out bed next to mine. During the night, we started discussing names. We hadn't thought that far ahead but all of a sudden were faced with that decision. I asked him what American Football players had played for both the Detroit Lions (which he supports) as well as the Minnesota Vikings (my team). We looked it up and a couple of names came up, but Riley (Reiff, #71) stuck out. Riley. Just saying it out loud felt good. When the miscarriage started, we weren't sure of the baby's gender so this was an excellent unisex choice as well.

Eventually, we fell asleep. The next morning, I got all checked out again to make sure my body was healing okay after labour and surgery. The medical team asked if we wanted to do an autopsy, to see what had happened and give them an opportunity to research more into stillborn births. About 1 in 8 pregnancies end in miscarriage so it is very common (www.nhs.uk). I have always been pro-science and tried to make sure medical technologies can advance so I said 'yes'. For myself, I wanted to make sure it was not Lupus that had caused the stillbirth (even with an eye to any potential future pregnancies). I signed off on the autopsy and was allowed to go back home to Rotterdam to recover.

I was given their official documentation so that I could get an official death certificate because even though he was only 18 weeks, he was very loved and I wanted to make sure he was properly registered and remembered.

Two days went by when I got the phone call, that I could pick up his body. It was Monday morning. My mother, our three year old son and I were about to bring my partner back to Schiphol Airport as he couldn't take any more work days off. After dropping him off, we went on to Amsterdam City Council to register Riley's death. It was very strange being back in the centre of the city I loved so much, where I lived for years before moving to Ireland in 2013. Familiar, but due to the recent events, I also felt strangely disconnected to everything. My brain was in survival mode.

When we arrived at the morgue connected to the hospital, Riley was laid out beautifully. All bandaged up because of the autopsy, but his face was as handsome as ever. Candles all around, his baby hospital band on the side table next to him. We had a little casket ready for him and because of my love for the ocean, I had bought him an octopus teddy. Moving his body into the little casket is by far the weirdest and most painful thing I had ever done.

We went to Rotterdam, this time with my 3 year old son and his little brother in the casket. I had rung the funeral home in advance. I wanted to get him cremated so I could take his ashes home with me to Ireland. Back to my stoic self, I got all the paperwork sorted and they asked if I wanted to bring him down to the cremator so I could send him off. I told my son to say goodbye to his baby brother and I carried Riley down the stairs.

Back upstairs, the funeral director told me I could pick up the ashes after a couple of days. Legal procedures in the Netherlands mean they would have to keep the ashes for 1 month, but they knew I was flying home to Ireland. He had a letter ready for me to sign to ask the public prosecutor for exemption in releasing the ashes.

By the end of the week I had another phone call, this time that we could pick up Riley's ashes. It was the same funeral director greeting us when we got to the crematorium, and again he had everything ready I needed to sign. He had also included an official letter for the airline that I had ashes and I had permission to fly with them.

Another bizarre revelation. I was supposed to go on holidays, have a good time with my son at my mother's mobile home before the baby got here. I wasn't supposed to lose my baby and spend the first two weeks grieving and stressed about everything that had happened and needed to get done. Medically for me, Riley and all the paperwork that comes with death. As I flew home, I told the security at the airport I was flying with his ashes and asked if he needed to see the paperwork. The guard could see I was close to tears as I said that, shook his head and just told me to put the bag in the tray. A gentle word, and off to the gate I went.

At home in Ireland I could finally relax. Grieve. I took proper time for myself, to make sure my physical and mental health would get back up to par. Spent time with my son, told him what had happened in the best age-appropriate way I could. After a couple of weeks, the autopsy results came back. It wasn't Lupus, it was a freak accident that had caused the stillbirth. Nothing I could do about it, and nothing the medical world could have done to prevent it. I'm glad it wasn't my Lupus and could look on into the future with hope.

In October, I found out I was pregnant again. There was Hope. I was also absolutely terrified that there would be another stillbirth. There was a lot of extra care (and a lot of extra scans for them to keep track of my baby's health, but also for my anxiety) from my doctor here in Ireland during my pregnancy. My healthy rainbow baby, a daughter, was born July 2019.

Tips for Millennials dealing with Miscarriage and Stillbirth

There are child bereavement services (like rouwrijk.nl - who also does counselling in English) and trained bereavement nurses in the hospital. Talk to them. Talk. Share your story. A lot of people have gone through this, know that you are not alone. Speak your baby's name. Journal your story. Make sure you give yourself time to grieve. Grief doesn't happen in a straight line, it's up and down with good days and bad days and horrible days.

Practice mindfulness, in whatever ways work for you.

- Legal procedures ashes: https://www.rijksoverheid.nl/wetten-en-regelingen/productbeschrijvingen/ontheffing-bewaartermijn-asbus
- Statistics: https://www.nhs.uk/conditions/miscarriage/

Reference

https://www.nhs.uk/conditions/miscarriage/

Would You Drive a Ferrari with No Breaks?

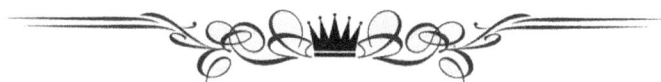

Louise Barry

"Living in the fast lane is great, as long as you remember where the slip roads are."

—Benny Bellamacina

As I journey down the road of life, I begin to wonder if my norm i.e., how I see the world is the same as my peers, family, friends and colleagues. I have had noticeable issues with my health from the age of 20 on, or at least that is when my frustration with issues such as memory, energy and organisational skills began.

This is when the direct consequences of these challenges were more seriously impacting my life. It would manifest itself in areas such as forgetting passwords and basic processing steps within my job. I was told after a period of absence from work that it was chronic fatigue by a specialist consultant who wasn't sure, but said that in all probability, I was evidently burnt out. This burn out was caused by sensory issues like sounds associated with too many people talking loudly around me, temperature changes in the room at work, distractions from other people asking me questions and interrupting my train of thought whilst I was working on something else. This all contributed to my fatigue at the end of a day at work causing me to be overwhelmed and resulting in my ultimate absence from work. He added, that hopefully, the underlying cause would reveal itself one day. That was 20 years ago. Knowing now, that these symptoms were all associated with ADHD has been a massive relief for me.

Since then, I have had bouts of anxiety, mild depression, and issues with my blood sugar. Doctors were mystified by what was organically happening to me. My attitude remained mainly positive which was helped largely by the support of my peers. Remaining hopeful, I pushed through but never unearthed why I was sometimes going through this myriad of issues. I seemed to have a boom-and-bust experience. I had great jobs, but I couldn't keep up with all the paperwork. I put this down to dyslexia in combination with my poor organisational skills.

I soldiered on and found myself at home in front of a mic and writing music when I was aged 30. In this space, I was free. All that was required of me, was living in the 'here and now'. No one to answer to but myself at my own pace. My creative spirit and space to breathe.

Since the last chapter I wrote in collaboration with Giselle Marrinan in Mental Health for Millennials4 (2020) my life has turned 180 degrees. Do I still agree with what I shared? What has happened since then? In this interim period, I contracted Covid-19 with delta variant symptoms. I collapsed at home and because I was living alone, I was taken via ambulance to Waterford Regional Hospital. Here, I was treated and kept in the intensive care unit for two weeks. I had trouble breathing and was unable to walk. I knew I had to entrust my life to the health care team to whom I'll be eternally grateful. They saved my life and protected me in my then vulnerable state.

Since then, I've had to simplify everything. I re-evaluated my life; what was important for me and what survival skills I had already.

- A warm home

- Clean bed
- Nutritious food
- Learning to ask for help
- Self-care
- Finding my inner resilience within the most difficult of circumstances
- I've grown in courage and strength during this difficult health crisis and know now that I can bounce back from anything

During this time, I received an email out of the blue saying, "Hi sis". It was from a gentleman who advised me that he was my oldest brother on my father's side of the family. Apparently, he had been given up for adoption years ago. He entered my life with love and generosity, courage and strength. He was open to the relationship which might develop between himself and his long-lost half-sister. Both, he, and his family have been a blessing to me and I'm very grateful for this experience at this stage in my life.

Diagnosis ADHD

Over time, a lot of things are becoming clear to me about my family history. In particular, the knowledge of health issues. One was related to blood sugar / diabetic issues and ADHD (Attention, Deficit, Hyperactivity, Disorder).

My brother very kindly remarked that, perhaps, I was also ADHD. It was a bit of sibling bantering but as time went on, I wondered whether, he may have been serious about the link. According, to the NHS website (2022), *"ADHD tends to run in families, and, in most cases, it's thought the genes you inherit from your parents are a significant factor in developing the condition"*.

169

Could This Be a Light Bulb Moment?

I researched the symptoms associated with ADHD and was shocked to find an exact description of what had been happening to me through the years. I went to see my GP and he also commented on my creativity, anxiety and depression. He confirmed that, it was something worth looking into. What a light bulb moment at the age of 42, to finally discover what has been holding me back in many areas of my life but also what has been a driving force in my creativity. As they say in the ADHD community, *"You are a Ferrari with no brakes."* Seemingly, many people with ADHD, find themselves in occupations where risk taking and being able to evaluate things from a broad perspective comes under their list of strengths and therefore become useful attributes within their careers. People like Richard Branson (Dean 2014), Elon Musk and Albert Einstein, to name but a few. Also, many musicians such as Mick Fleetwood and Cher, artists such as Pablo Picasso and Vincent van Gogh, and stylists like Crystal Casey too. I hear it said within the ADHD community that, it is not that there is something wrong with us but just, that the world is set up to work for people with non-neurotypical brains.

Having recently spoken to my psychiatrist about medication, he articulated what the impact of this might have on the creative side of my work. This concerned him. He suggested we keep the parts of the ADHD that are driving forces, like my inventive thinking, creativity and my ability to hyperfocus - sticking with a job until it is finished and an actual positive attribute whilst still trying to help me to deal with the fact that I'm not making enough dopamine in my brain to have a great working memory. I am blessed by his forward-thinking and this has given me real hope about my new future.

ADHD and the Strengths Attributed to It

On the ADHD Ireland website (2022), under 'Shine a Light', I watched a video about different individuals experiences with ADHD. Bryn Travers stated that the strengths he would keep from his disorder would include:

1. Creativity
2. Excess energy levels
3. Spontaneity – ability to improvise on the spot

So, What Are My Strengths and How Have I Used These in the Music Industry?

One of my strengths is the ability to hyper focus, meaning that when I concentrate on one thing, I give all my energy to it zoning out of everything else around me. I am so consumed with the music and the ensuing ideas that flow from them, that everything else just melts away, sometimes for hours at a time.

Because of all the challenges thrown my way over the years, I occasionally thought, "Why me?". I wanted to be like other people's families being able to organise things – organising papers, relationships etc. But there has been a recent paradigm shift. Instead of asking. "Why me?", I say, "Why not me?" I can stand back from my life and see that for every challenge I have encountered, my personal growth has increased exponentially. My generous and spontaneous spirit helps me to say yes to things which others would be more fearful of.

Despite and because of these challenges, I am being moulded into a more resilient person. I am gaining wisdom and understanding of my condition and working in harmony with my strengths. I try not to take myself too seriously and am now able to laugh at my short comings. This has helped me during darker periods of my life where my quirky little ways can light up the more serious challenges which I have encountered.

I am becoming more empathetic, using my wealth of experience to advocate for others who have mental health issues. My passion lies in wanting to support others in their endeavours and indeed I seem to be the person people come to, to find an alternative way to look at their creative projects and interpersonal problems.

My Weaknesses and How I Overcome Them

If there is a weakness with my condition, it is that I don't understand the concept of time. I can procrastinate and forget to reach out to people in my life. I always tell people that if I don't contact them, reach out to me, and nudge me into action. But, because I am so good at living in the moment, in the now, that when I am with people, involved with projects or in certain places, I am totally engaged.

I have even managed to deal with distractions whilst performing live as something as small as a flashlight from a photographer can halt my train of thought and I lose my spot in the song. This happened once to me, where the light blinded me, and I became completely overwhelmed. Whilst processing this, I lost my place in the song and had to listen carefully to the band to pick it up again. This was totally unnerving and made me incredibly anxious but, as we say in the business, "the show must go on" and when I could concentrate on the band again, I just picked up the song again. These moments on stage can feel like an eternity and I must be careful not to beat myself up about this later. My musicians are great at handling these lapses since they know my weaknesses and are ready to support me. They give a trigger in the music to let me know where we are in a song.

Hope for Others with ADHD

These last few years, I have been lucky enough to be able to share my experiences at many levels and on different forums. I have been a guest speaker at national schools, at UCC, UCD, featured in the national press and radio. I have also been recently aired on Keith Russell's multi- award nominated mental health awareness and wellbeing podcast, "The Endless Spiral". I am telling you this, not to boast but to encourage you to live a life without limitations. A diagnosis is just the beginning of your journey.

This volume has as its themes, hope and inclusion. I intend to continue working as a mental health advocate to give others strength and hope for the future. Hope is the gentlest of things.

Tips for Coping with ADHD

- Organising your time – Use technology like Google calendar as an aide memoir.
- When you feel stress coming up, ensure periods of good quality rest. Practice a lot of loving kindness towards yourself.
- Try walking to calm the mind and body.
- Monitor your diet. Certain foods will engage with your ADHD instead of bringing you out of balance. Although the research on nutrition for ADHD is varied, there is no doubt that, *"you're eating habits would help the brain work better and lessen symptoms, such as restlessness or lack of focus"* (Roybal 2021).
- Enjoy animals, kids, the arts, and life in general. Be a part of life.
- Keep your sense of humour. When you feel emotionally overwhelmed with feelings of rejection or sensitivity, lessen your exposure to social media and watch comedy.

- Stay informed. Read about ADHD.

- Listen to podcasts which encourage you particularly from those who are walking a similar path.

- Group support like ADHD Adult support helps hold a mirror up to your own personal way of being, coping mechanisms and indeed giftedness. It is encouraging to meet like-minded people.

- Have an ADHD buddy who can support you when the going gets tough.

- Meditation is key to being grounded and finding a healthy baseline of well-being.

- Remember self- awareness is growing into yourself. Self-acceptance is the greatest love you can experience.

You have only one body mind and soul. Nourish it.

In Conclusion

One of the best things about my being finally diagnosed, is that I am getting better at understanding my brain's abilities and when I need to ask for support. I am learning that I am unique and yes different, but instead of being afraid or hiding from it, I am learning to embrace and channel it through creative mediums. In this, I see great inclusion.

I am challenging myself to be imperfect and still perfectly lovable. I have identified the slip roads. There is hope for all of us.

I wish to thank my ghost writer, Giselle Marrinan, who worked closely with me in the telling of my story.

References

Barry, L. (2020) Mental Health for Millennials. On Wellbeing. Vol 4. 'Music & Wellbeing'. Book Hub Publishing, Galway.

www.nhs.uk/conditions/attention-deficit-hyperactivity-disorder-dhd/causes/#:~:text=Genetics, likely%20to%20have%20ADHD%20themselves

Dean, T. "You'd Never Guess These Famous People Had ADHD". News24.com. Jul 2014.

https://adhdireland.ie/shine-a-light-understanding-adhd-video/

Roybal, B. "ADHD Diet and Nutrition: Foods to Eat and Foods to Avoid" WebMed June 2021.

Inclusion in Sport and Coaching

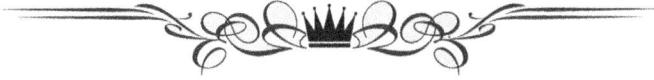

Thomas Kiely

Introduction

My hope for the future of inclusion in sport and coaching is that the importance of local rural and community sports clubs will be enhanced. Perhaps not many people realise the importance of having these clubs in rural areas, especially since Covid-19 arrived on our doorsteps in 2020. Sport gives parents, children, and coaches *hope* that there is some bit of normality coming back into our lives and, that it will remain. The anxiety, fear and the unknown during Covid times have brought another negative dimension to people's lives that they hadn't experienced previously, so having a rural/local club has perhaps helped these people out some bit, and I think the importance of this isn't spoken about as much as it should in terms of the themes of this book; inclusion and hope.

As a coach in my local rural club, seeing regular participation of anything between 30 to 40 children of all different ages was fantastic, considering how small a club we are—seeing the excitement in these children's faces just kicking a ball and with coaches' help, learning something new every night is wonderful. For these children and parents alike, the talk of Covid isn't mentioned too much by us; the coaches. However, we did take every precautionary measure to make sure we have a safe place for the children.

I, as a coach, wanted the children to enjoy the training sessions and that they learned something new each time they attended my sessions. I wanted them to arrive and leave with a sense of hope in their hearts.

Children are in school/ pre-school throughout the day, so for me, the importance for the children is the enjoyment of their involvement. I always mentioned how I wanted the children to be happy coming down to training. They actually enjoyed it. Also, I wanted the connection with children that they feel they could ask any questions, and if they weren't happy, they could approach me as a coach. If a parent needed to ask questions, we were available for them. My hope for the future is for more children to become and, crucially, stay involved in sport, and I will return to this point shortly. The involvement of parents is also significant in the future of our club and, indeed, any club.

As mentioned in my last paragraph, my hope is for more children to stay involved in sports for so many reasons, and here are some of them.

The social and communication aspect. For children, getting out in the open and meeting classmates' friends or making new friends is so essential for their development in life in general. It will give them confidence growing up and further enhance their ability to express themselves and ask questions and not be afraid to hope for the best for themselves in the future. The importance of children expressing themselves is very important, whether this is on the training field or on match days. It gives them confidence that maybe I didn't have at their age.

Life Dangers

Nowadays, we live in a world with so much uncertainty and dangers for children growing up. The hope for parents is that their children stay out of trouble, either with drugs alcohol or fall into a group that leads them to get into domestic trouble. I believe that the local sports clubs give parents hope that the children with the help of us the coaches guide them in the right direction, what I mean in regards guide them, well with team sports it's important that the children understand that we are all together as a team. We all look after our teammates whether they have an off day at training or maybe something important happened in their lives, then the teammates are there for each other. The hope for me is with the enjoyment in training and having ground rules that the children will take on board and stay involved longer in sports and the future teams in the club.

The importance of my local sports club has helped me massively on a personal note. I sadly lost my wife, Angela, in November 2019. She was 33. I was only briefly involved in the club in the background, just helping out with my son's team, but when Angela died, I got more involved with training myself and training the kids. I also helped out more and became assistant club secretary thereby getting involved in the administration of sending out details for the underage training groups to organising games, setting up training and always trying to improve the club's underage setup.

I hope that someone that has, or maybe is going through, hard times considers getting involved in club life. Reconnecting with other parents has helped me massively; it gave me an outlet, it allowed me to switch off for the few hours that I was down coaching, and I enjoyed watching the children have fun and being able to express themselves, which is so essential for me.

My hope for the future of the local club is to get more parents involved in the rural club scene. There is a fear around getting involved in coaching, and there shouldn't be. In coaching, some of the children feel like they have to know everything about their sport, but in reality, they don't as they will have the consistent help of a coach. Everyone is involved. We all go home happy and that is why the parental involvement is key.

To get more parents involved in the club, we also need more coaches, which from a small rural/local club is a difficult task, so the hope in the future is to get maybe players that are playing now or former players that can bring some new ideas into the general setup where roles can be allocated and distributed across the age ranges. I think the satisfaction of watching children develop weekly, monthly and yearly gives everyone great enjoyment and the feeling that we are doing something meaningful, so hopefully, in the future, our small club will have more parents and coaches involved.

Sport is for All

My final hope for our local club is the get more children with learning difficulties or any other issues they might have more involved. For a small rural club to have this option available for local parents would be fantastic. It would save the parents so much financially with travelling to other parts of the county and let local parents get together and be genuinely involved in the club's day to day life which is the heartbeat of a local community. I think the club would benefit massively as with so many illnesses, learning difficulties and lack of local amenities for these people, it will show that the club wants to reach out to and help the local community and parents.

Take Away Nuggets

- Sport is for everyone.
- Sport should, first and foremost, be fun.
- Coaches are hugely meaningful to a club's overall longevity.
- Rural communities need their local clubs for a sense of identity and community.

Thomas recently moved to the UK but maintains an active interest in his local club.

Creating a Sense of Hope in the Swirling World of the Metaverse and Social Media 'Beautification'

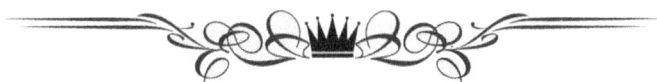

Elaine De Roiste

"It's not my place in society that makes me well off, but my judgments; and these I can carry with me... These alone are my own and cannot be taken away"

— (Epictetus, Discourses, (c. AD 100).

Introduction: Setting the Context

I am seeing increasing levels of unhappiness, loneliness and a deep longing for inclusion across social media despite the fact that people have access to so much technology, connectedness and (potential) immediacy (Srivastava and Chandra, 2018). Why might this be? Why do so many need validation and acceptance? Is loneliness the new post Covid epidemic? What might be behind it all? Why are so many people so unhappy and, crucially, where is the(ir) hope.

Elaine De Roiste

In the western world, we live in an era characterised by hypermodernity, hyper consumerism and hyper narcissism. Perhaps the human species has always been this way (there's certainly no shortage of statues from the ancient world) and it is just technology that better facilitates the expression of this.

Indeed, we are used to smartphones, iPhones and tablets recording events in real time and social media ensures 'followers' and virtual 'friends' get to share our beautified and filtered experiences in nano seconds. Could this be our new reality, our new home? A place where we are always winning but no one posts their failures. While we are busy in our online world, when are we 'present', here. Is our 'here' or reality so intolerable or lonely we need the escape and the constant validation of strangers. Our new online audience, our online friends who, too, don't seem to be present. But we believe that all of this 'demand for expression and validation' is having an increasingly negative effect on the development and expression of positive self-esteem and on the potential development of pervasive social anxiety for individuals. For all too many, it is interfering with their sense of a hopeful future. For many, it limits the actual ability to connect and be present in real life. We lose the ability to simply chat, to speak, to connect. Let's face it. Connection is the goal. It's the highway to *more*. More than validation, connection is really where it's at. However, more, in this case, is not always a good thing.

The world's population is predicted to reach 9.3bn by 2050 but there are vast differences in terms of standards of living between various regions of the world. Mass communication is now everyday reality and Ireland has the highest rate of smartphone usage per capita in western Europe. Facebook, Linked In, and Instagram, to name but three platforms, are at our fingertips and we can upload and share our (filtered) photos, in real time. And, yes, I am on all these platforms before you ask

☺. Is this where our lives are 'at' now. Is this our reality or our escape?

Is this ubiquitous social media presence and online existence for us all (Thies, Wessel and Benlian, 2016) a positive thing? I'm going to say, simply, 'no'. I don't think so. In fact, I would argue that more time in the real world is the only effective antidote to life on social media. There is nothing quite like meeting a real person in the physical world for a real conversation, connection, eye contact. Are we now losing that ability because we spend so much time on our phones that we are never present, never connecting. The simple hello is somewhat lost online. Online we can be whomever we choose. We can hide. And we do, don't we? Wait. What about the biggest hiding place of them all. The 'metaverse' I hear you ask...

A Few Words on the Metaverse

Interestingly, the metaverse dates back to 1992 and was first mentioned by sci-fi writer, Neal Stephenson, in the novel Snow Crash. We are talking vast finances here as it's now projected to be worth some 760millionUSD in less than five years from now, and Meta, Microsoft, and Google have all announced plans to create new virtual worlds (Zhadan, 2022).

The metaverse and Web3 are now catch-all terms that describe various aspects of what is perceived to be the future Internet (Di Pietro and Cresci, 2021). But, it's important to know that technologies are constructing immersive worlds that, to greater and lesser extents, intersect digital and real life. More and more people are migrating to the metaverse to work, play and 'live,' but we are clueless as to what this really means in terms of sense of self and identity (Bourgi, 2022). Will it bring more or less hope to people as individuals? Let's not forget that, amongst lots of other businesses and platforms, Meta owns Facebook, Instagram, and WhatsApp. We are all part of the(ir) global empire.

Yogesh et al (2022) make the point that impacted sectors include marketing, education, healthcare as well as societal effects relating to social interaction factors from widespread adoption, and issues relating to trust, privacy, bias, disinformation, application of law as well as psychological aspects linked to addiction and impact on vulnerable people. There's a lot going on there!

Conclusion

We quickly learn rewarded and unrewarded behaviours and usually (although not always) modify our behaviour as we are, in essence, a pleasure seeking (as opposed to pain!) species. Hence, if we get a negative comment on a photo we post, we can immediately go back into our post, refilter the photo and present a new image. An altered image just like an altered reality. A better image of us. A more socially accepted, more clicks, more validation. When does it become real that this isn't real and neither is our behaviour? We are all flawed this is true. Uniquely and beautifully flawed. Presenting a version of ourselves online that we can't present in real life actually removes us further from any possible reality or genuine connection.

Imagine then how our self-esteem can grow and mature if we actively choose to engage with positive, like-minded people who, of course, challenge us in the real world or the world of the metaverse. Imagine how our feelings of hope and sense of inclusion can grow when we feel our relationships are mutually reciprocal. Imagine being present and saying "this is me, freckles and all".

I wish to thank my ghost writer, Dr. Niall MacGiolla Bhuí, who worked closely with me in writing this chapter.

References

Di Pietro, R., and Cresci, S. (2021). "Metaverse: Security and Privacy Issues", The Third IEEE International Conference on Trust, Privacy and Security in Intelligent Systems, and Applications, December 13-15, 2021.

Srivastava, S. C., and Chandra, S. (2018). "Social presence in virtual world collaboration: An uncertainty reduction perspective using a mixed methods approach", MIS Quarterly, Vol. 42 No.3, pp. 779-804.

Thies, F., Wessel, M., and Benlian, A. (2016). "Effects of social interaction dynamics on platforms", Journal of Management Information Systems, Vol. 33 No. 3, pp. 843-873.

Yogesh K. et l., (2022). Metaverse beyond the hype: Multidisciplinary perspectives on emerging challenges, opportunities, and agenda for research, practice and policy, International Journal of Information Management, Volume 66, 2022, 102542, ISSN 0268-4012, https://doi.org/10.1016/j.ijinfomgt.2022.102542.

URL Articles

Bourgi, S (2022). https://cointelegraph.com/news/the-dark-side-of-the-metaverse-and how-to-fight-it-cointelegraph-interview Accessed September 2nd 2022.

Zhadan, A. (2022).

https://cybernews.com/editorial/the-dark-side-of-the-metaverse-taking-your-nightmar es-online/ Accessed September 1st 2022.

Creative Writing

Nocturnal

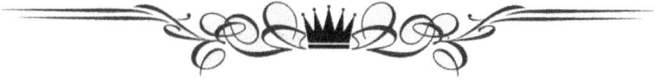

Edel Hanley

Tonight memories walk memory lane with us,
holding our heads as if to guide us by something other than our hands.
Why is it that they always forget to warn us of the past,
the past that swoops down, like nightly terrors or dark predators,
to grab hold of your shirt as if they were all the person
you didn't want to become?
Inside I wrote a letter telling you all about it
but just the thought of you is enough to keep me up.
I am nocturnal, you see, even in the day that's breaking.

Act of Contrition

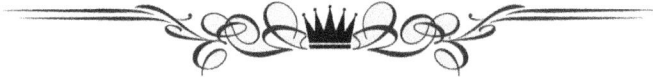

Edel Hanley

On the day of the wake I hid a rosary of rainbow beads
inside your palm
because they might have been the only thing
you'd have to remember me
when you woke on the other side.
I wonder if you have it still,
planted carefully at your ribcage,
its peas of plastic seeding your bones
to grow the garden you once had in life –
cabbages, lettuce, parsnips and cherry tomatoes.
As a child I pulled these with my very own hands
and passed them to you.
That was the year of I had my very first Act of Contrition.

Love Poem

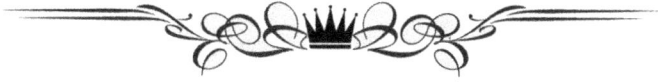

Edel Hanley

If you don't love me, I promise not to love you, either.
And I won't say anything as if it's anything at all.
Instead I'll pluck the past like wilted leaves
and remember that love will spring again
when the birds return to eat what's left of us.

TAP TAP TIPPY TIPPY TAP

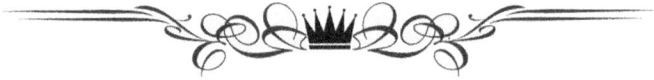

Giovanni Mangiante

You are by the edge of the bed, licking your right paw. One of your
nails is broken.
I watch, fading in and out, half a whiskey bottle on the desk.
Tchaikovsky's Waltz of The Flowers plays on the computer.
We haven't played in months.
You wait. You bring your green chewing plastic bone, I throw it away.
You bring it back, but I'm not laughing.
You go back towards the edge of the bed and lick your paw.
You would like to clasp your jaws on the throat of whatever possesses me,
but it's just me there slumped over.
Some time ago, I was fit and we both played for hours. I was fast.
I carried you around the house on one arm. I was strong.
My body shut down three times in the last two months, but I won't go
to the doctor.
"I'm alright" I say, and you hear the clinking of ice cubes from the
kitchen again.
You go. I give you one. I drown them in bitter caramel and I sink.
Deep underwater you kick with your paws, downwards, downwards,
downwards,
and catch me by the shirt with your mouth. You swim up, up, up.
You forget your broken nail, and you lick my face instead.
I touch your ear.

I'M SURE THERE IS A GOOD REASON

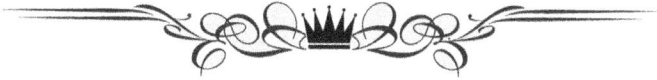

Giovanni Mangiante

The coffee marches inside my stomach
while I think of how alone it feels
being inside this room
with no one to love, smoking a cigarette
and pissing.
I throw ashes inside the toilet bowl,
take another hit of the cigarette.
I knew there had to be something waiting
to make itself real.
Not just this waiting. Not just this longing.
I thought about my mother, father, sister,
dog, nonna, friends, my guitar catching dust
in the corner of the room,
the piles of books I so eagerly bought,
the new job I'd start in the next two weeks,
and I realized I hadn't felt like dying
in two years despite the downfalls.
I took another hit of the cigarette and
saw the ashes floating inside the bowl.
There was a reason. I had gotten the upper hand
in the fight.

UP

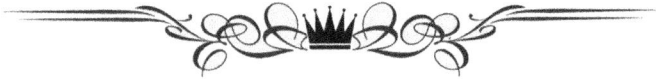

Giovanni Mangiante

I'm not the bloody bandages
I left behind
nor the blades I attempted
to shred myself off from
earth with.

I'm my father's luminescent smile
when we have dinner
and I'm sober.

I'm not the blood.
I'm not the bottle.
I'm not the victim.

I'm the flower
looking at the concrete
wall
from underneath
the ground,
knowing
there is only one way
out of it.

Up.

Speaking of the Doves

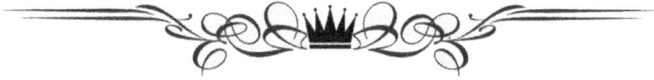

John Ennis

Our dovecote high above the battlements,
We look down on the defenders of the realm.
We rule the roost and just our coos
Are visible as the night it cuddles in at Fore.

There is always a beginning and an end to things,
From the foundation stones of the cote on a morning
When the sun it must have shone, such hopes
For our wings still fluttering across millennia.

Don't underestimate us ever, the doves,
If on all sides we're the dove-trodden,
Our dovecote fallen. Listen out for us
As the memories of oak leaves cease.

Where the Grey Crow Feeds with the Sparrow

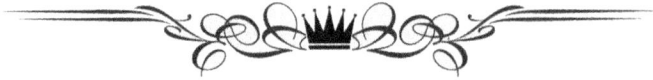

John Ennis

Dropping down you take the bones left out,
the bones of your feathered kind, for one
finds chicken mostly in *Cirrabiata* takeaways.
On two concrete pillars resting butt to butt:
I didn't know what to do with those pillars
that opened out once into the outer haggard
where the corn stacks waited for John Harte:
chaff after him, lots of corn flowers, *praiseach*
bees go crazy for. So, twin altars for you both
to feed on, in frost, or times of luxuriance
of stem. The close ivied sparrows alight first
chorusing their luck toward the noon-day sun's
bigger cousins. Crows, magpies, scald crows
dancing about the morsels too, broken bones.

Assumption Eve

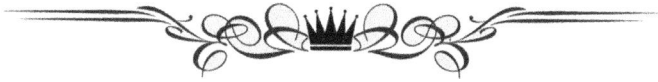

John Ennis

The last Assumption eve I saw them together
My mother, Jack, and my father,
Mid-August evening, a dry spell.
Down from the new bungalow, the old man's drills
Of cabbage plants newly in, they could do
With a watering. And Jack is doing this
While the three are laughing at something
All still to the good, hale, if ageing, as I
Step out of the car. Tony has picked me up
In Maynooth. I'm home on my last break
Before the Masters. The plants are thriving,
Why wouldn't they be, the clay and mould of thatch
With bog scraw where the roof fell in a few years back.
And we are in no hurry at all to break the magic
Of the twilight, Jack watering, the old man at ease
For once, outside, and my mother talking to her brother
Uplifted above the unimportant, as Jack he fills his last
Bucket from the tank he built, the plants are well soaked now.

In Memory of William Corbally

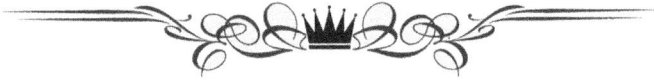

John Ennis

i

Some morning I must drive up to Cruicetown
to read that slab of a poem
someone wrote for a father's son
in whom the latter might have been well pleased
had he not pre-deceased him by twenty-six years

William Corbally

who was late of Drogheda, a merchant
the recollection of whose many virtues
will be very cherished by a numerous
and respectable circle of acquaintances
and must prove a source of melancholy
consolation to his afflicted friends
he exchanged his temporal for eternal life
on 5th April 1827 in the 30th year of his age . . .

seems like the life and soul of the party
walked out on the thirtieth year of his heaven like DT
friends gathered round his smooth slab of limestone in a roofless
church
a Phlebas of his day, a Myras of the late hours, who knows
seems he just slipped away, not much of a surprise
and what William was merchant of we do not know

save his father George never got to see his son blossom dying himself at
51
in 1801, the year Will's sister Catherine died at nine, no word of
spouse or kids
but William has the lion's share on that south slab, his orientation is
east-west,
the rest eternal rest
and every time the sky it rains on it, the flat black limestone shines
maybe I'll be lucky the mid-morning I call to find the heavens opening
over him
the rain drops dancing on the black limestone.

ii
around him useless errata of a bye-gone age
the church building blocks that lost out with King James
five stones in a row, our place for sure, these grave markers

the Board of Works removed the supports for all table tombs
the living can walk safer now, but imagine all that weight
on your breast bone waiting for the trumpet of belief

moulds of door or stone window jamb arch for a door or window
the mortar still hanging on
good concrete that

with other older slabs whose names are unintelligible
but these may not be names at all
just tool markings of apprentices
still

shine for us eternally William Corbally
young merchant from Drogheda

Braiden Jacob

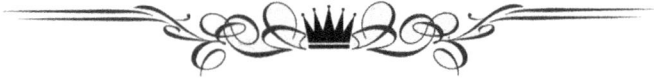

John Ennis

What's another boy in Thunder Bay
Just another post from *Fiddler News*
Never knew him, or of him, that boy,
His kind, save he dies in Thunder Bay

Needs counselling, and who does not
Hope a star shone for him on his own
Those last moments in Chapples Park
Across the long ways in Thunder Bay

So it is our sunlit coming, our going
Thunder or none in no Thunder Bay,
Remember him when you next hear
That crash up in your own heavens

Whisper his name soft so he'll hear,
Braiden Jacob, so he'll open his eyes
Laugh again, in whatever community
There is, this side now or the other.

(a note of context)

Braiden Jacob's body was found Sunday in Thunder Bay.

Willow Fiddler
APTN News

The body found on a Thunder Bay golf course late Sunday morning is that of a missing 17-year-old youth, the chief of Webequie First Nation confirmed.

Chief Cornelius Wabasse told *APTN News* the family met with police around 7:45 p.m. Sunday.

"The forensic team came in first and then the coroner called to reaffirm that it was Braiden, the body that was found this morning," said Wabasse.

Braiden Jacob was reported missing Dec. 6.

His family had last seen him on Wednesday night when he left the hotel they were staying in. They started searching for him when he didn't return later that night.

Community volunteers began an organized search for the missing teen on Thursday afternoon.

The youth was in the city for ongoing counselling services for trauma and grief, according to Wabasse.

"They're very distraught, I mean it's very emotional. Not just with the family but the extended family too," he said.

"Even the community is impacted by the loss of a young man."

Jacob was from Webequie, a fly-in community approximately 600 km north of Thunder Bay.

On Saturday, Thunder Bay police released further details of Jacob's disappearance including a description of what he was wearing.

They said the youth was last seen in the early Thursday in the Limbrick area. His body was found on the golf course in Chapples Park less than 3 km away.

In a media release Sunday afternoon, police said they were dispatched to the park area around 11:30 a.m when a passerby reported a possible body.

It's the same park where Tammy Keeash was found drowned in the floodway that runs through the park May 2017 – and the body of 32-year-old William Wapoose was discovered in September 2014.

His homicide remains unsolved.

Anna Betty Achneepineskum of Nishnawbe Aski Nation expressed frustration on Facebook over the of health services available on-reserve.

"Why is it that we have to bring our children out to an urban centre to get counselling service?" said Achneepineskum.

"It's not right that we have a system that continues to jeopardize our children's safety."

Community members from Thunder Bay and other First Nations gathered on Sunday to offer support to Jacob's family and community.

The body has been taken to Toronto for a post-mortem.

wfiddler@aptn.ca

@WillowBlasizzo

About the Authors

Dr. Niall MacGiolla Bhuí was founding editor of the Irish Journal of Applied Social Studies and editor-in-chief at that journal for a decade. He has travelled extensively lecturing and presenting workshops across Ireland, Northern Ireland, England, Sweden and coast to coast Canada. Niall is series co-editor, along with Dr. Phil Noone, of the seven book series, Mental Health For Millennials (published by Book Hub Publishing and sponsored by the consulting agency TheDocChck.Com 2017-2023 - available in both paperback and downloadable eBook on Amazon). He is also founder and editor of the #ExploringConnectedness book series and the co-editor of this book. He has authored three books and co-authored another ten books with colleagues across various mental health and humanities themes. Niall currently ghostwrites for a range of national and international clients and mentors Masters and Doctoral candidates across the university sector. His second book of poetry will be published in 2023.

Dr. Phil Noone is a Mindfulness Coach/Lecturer with a nursing background who has travelled and worked extensively abroad in a variety of health and well-being settings. She holds an MSc in Mindfulness Based Interventions, a Diploma in Mindfulness and Positive Psychology, a PhD in Sociology and an MSc in Health Promotion. Phil has lectured for many years at the School of Nursing and Midwifery, University of Galway, and has presented at conferences in South America, Holland, Australia and Ireland. Phil is series co-editor and chapter contributor along with Dr Niall MacGiolla Bhuí of the Mental Health for Millennial Series (1-7), has published papers and conducted research on the themes of 'home', 'well-being', 'rural ageing', 'resilience', 'environmental action and sustainability' and 'Mindfulness'. She has recently set up her own business 'Ocean Mindfulness', delivering Mindfulness at corporate and community level.

Dr. Mary Helen Hensley is an internationally published author and a doctor of chiropractic. She was Book Hub Publishing's first published author back in 2009 and holds 'bestselling status.' Mary Helen is Head of Diversity, Inclusion and Equality at TheDocCheck.Com and regularly speaks and presents at international symposia and conferences where she is much sought after. She has published ten books and is a regular visitor to the United States where she consults to the stars of Broadway and LA and is involved in a range of writing projects.

Giselle Marrinan MSc holds an MSc in Applied Immunology and was a Fellow of The Institute of Biomedical Sciences. She was a sales director of an International Cancer Diagnostics company for whom she worked for 17 years. She has been an editor with this Series over the past three books, has contributed several chapters and is a ghost writer.

Susan McKenna B.A., Dip. Social Studies is Director of Book Hub Publishing where she is Commissioning Editor and Author Rep. She graduated in social care with a first class degree and has over two decades experience in social care practice and management. Susan is a former Erasmus Scholar (Stockholm) and Lectured p/t in Waterford and Athlone Institutes of Technology in addition to presenting workshops in east and west coast Canada. She has written widely on social care themes and is the co-author of two books in addition to having published several chapters in Book Hub Hub's Mental Health for Millennials Series (2017-2023).

Daragh Fleming MSc is an author from Cork in Ireland who uses a conversational style to delve into complex themes which emerge in everyday life. He runs an award-nominated mental health blog and is active voice for mental health in Ireland, delivering talks in a variety of schools, universities and work places. He has two collections of short stories published by Riversong Books, as well as two poetry pamphlets published. His most recent pamphlet, 'Poems That Were Written On Trains But Weren't Written About Trains' was released in July of 2022. His debut in nonfiction – 'Lonely Boy' - arrives with Book Hub Publishing in November 2022.

Anne Hayden MSc is a doctoral studies candidate in agricultural economics at University College Dublin, Ireland. She holds a Master of Science from the UCD Michael Smurfit Graduate Business School in Food Business Strategy and a Bachelor in Agricultural Science. Her research interests are the environmental, social and economic regional impacts of possible policy changes to the common agricultural policy. Anne has been a guest contributor to Mental Health for Millennials Volume 5 (2021) on the theme of resilience in Irish agriculture and Mental Health for Millennials Volume 6 (2022) on #hope for women in Irish agriculture. She has also been featured as a contributor in the TheDocCheck.Com published college studies series with her debut book.

Cathy Fitzgibbon MSc is a sales and marketing professional in the media industry for the past three decades. She is passionate about exploring contemporary culinary experiences and actively promotes the areas of food sustainably and food tourism through her food writing contributions and marketing activities under her alias 'The Culinary Celt', using an ethically based farm to fork ethos. She has also contributed to several Book Hub Publishing books and TheDocCheck.Com publications in addition to presenting academic research papers both nationally and internationally. Cathy consults with The Dissertation Doctors clinic and most recently published her debut book, 'Eat With The Seasons'.

Jennifer Murphy MSc is a graduate of University of Limerick. Jennifer has worked for the past fourteen years in various Human Resources roles across several Retail, Manufacturing and Hospitality Sectors. A Highly strategic HR professional with a passion for Talent Management, Culture and Employment Legislation, she consults with TheDocCheck.Com in the area of HR and research perspectives and has contributed as a guest author in the recent series "Exploring Connectedness" and Mental Health for Millennials Vol 6. She is Director of The HR & Governance Suite.

Karen Gallen Dip Marketing is a proud mum to two beautiful children, one of which has additional needs and is a 'scoliosis warrior'. Karen's focus is to shine light on additional needs and is an advocate having recently been interviewed on national radio on the RTE Radio Drivetime programme on the theme of raising awareness on the range of 'other' difficulties facing parents of children with additional needs such as accommodation for hospital stays etc. She continues to be a support to other parents on online platforms by sharing her lived experience. Karen's contributions on this matter can be read in Volume V in the Mental Health for Millennials book series and in the upcoming Volume VI of the same series, both published by The Book Hub Publishing Group.

Ray Flannery Dip Policing is a Detective Garda based in Dublin with over 30 years' experience in policing. He is also a children's book author with three books published in the #MoanyMcMoan series. He has contributed to the last five books in the Mental Health For Millennials Series. Ray is a keen golfer, musician and GAA coach in his spare time.

Paul Kilgannon BEd is a Coach and Athlete Mentor, Author and Creator of The CARVER Coaching Framework which is used internationally across a number of sports and industries. He helps people build their Coaching World and consults with Sporting Organisations and Clubs, as well as Corporate Entities in the area of creating Learning and Performance Environments. He has a particular interest in Youth Sports Coaching and has spent his adult life coaching across all age groups.

Louise Barry is a singer-songwriter who trained at the prestigious Paul McCartney School LIPA. She has been featured on national and international radio. She has also written and produced for the stage, video games, and Art Installations and film -fx's. Louise is a published author in peer-reviewed books and passionately advocates for positive mental health as a public speaker.

Sinéad O'Malley MSc is a graduate of University of Galway. During her time in university, she enjoyed being a brand ambassador for TheDocCheck.com. Having just completed a postgraduate programme in Business and a Masters in Human Resource Management, Sinéad commenced her HR career in the non-profit sector as an Intern in March of 2022. Since then, she has become part of the Talent Acquisition team at one of the world's biggest and fastest growing Irish companies who manufacture and distribute leading safety wear, workwear and PPE. She is a previous contributor to this series where she written about the impact on her life after losing a close friend to suicide.

Aine Crosse is a mother to 7 children, 3 whom have autism and mitochondrial disease. She is also an author with Book Hub Publishing. In the last five years, Aine has published 2 books: All That We Never See: Our Journey With Autism and From Stormy Seas to Calmer Waters. Aine and her late husband Gerry, document their arduous journey of how they navigate the unscripted world of autism and mitochondrial disease. Aine has had to live with many ups and downs in the past 3 years as, the start of 2020, as Aine and Gerry's son was diagnosed with cancer at just 17 years old. Then the unthinkable happened to Aine and her children; just 4 months later, on the 17th of June, Aine lost the love of her life, her rock. Her children lost their father, their support. Gerry died suddenly with no warning. Since then, Aine has learned from having to fight the system for help for her children, to knowing that tomorrow isn't promised to any of us, that you must live for the now and love always. Aine was very happy to be asked to guest author on Mental Health for Millennials Vol. 6.

Anna Gray is a qualified counsellor and psychotherapist, working with adults from all walks of life. She is the Northern Ireland Senior Reviewer for Book Hub Publishing and works with clients as a mentor and editor. Anna has contributed to a number of Mental Health For Millennials books and published her own book, 'Coming Out Of The Dark' in 2018. She is passionate about helping authors to tell their stories in their own voice and to write a book they will be proud of.

Anne Marie Doyle MSc is a graduate of University of Limerick and University of Galway. Anne Marie has been employed as a primary school teacher for the past twenty years, while also working as a Deputy Principal for the past fourteen years. She has a special interest in inclusion in mainstream classrooms and completed studies in psychology, dyslexia, autism and childhood anxiety. An experienced professional who has spent fourteen years in a leadership capacity, Anne Marie facilitates team-building, communicating her school's vision and striving to empower staff and students.

John Madden M.A is a graduate of Athlone Institute of Technology, and holds an MA in Advanced Social Care. He has worked in several areas over the years; primarily in mental health but also within inclusion and integration. He is currently the lead for Ukrainian support for New Horizon, a volunteer-led charity enacted to assist with the care and support of displaced peoples fleeing war and persecution. He has featured in all volumes of the Mental Health for Millenials series as well as being a key asset for academic support for TheDocCheck.Com Having covered a myriad of subjects ranging from self-harm to help-seeking. This chapter sees him explore the topic of recovery, which is dear to his heart as he also facilitates recovery support groups for a national mental health organisation.

Chris Sherlock is a Galway native, Broadcaster, Author and Anti-Bullying campaigner. From a young age, Chris has always had a huge passion for broadcasting, having started out in his early teens on internet radio, followed by working with Galway's College Radio station Flirt FM 101.3 (National University of Ireland). His best known feature is his C.S.I Sessions which are in-depth interviews that can be found on his radio show or as a podcast across the usual podcast platforms under "Chris Sherlock on the Wireless." Chris made his debut as an author in the book series Mental Health for Millennials Vol.4 (Book Hub Publishing 2020) where he contributed a chapter titled "A victim impact statement on being bullied at school" which explains his personal experience of being bullied at secondary school in Ireland. Since then, Chris features regularly in the press and on various radio stations raising bullying awareness. He makes a regular contribution to this aim by giving school talks and working with some organizations which work to end bullying in its various forms. Through this he has become an active anti-bullying campaigner. Chris has returned as a guest author in Mental

Health for Millennials Vol.6 (Book Hub Publishing 2022) with his chapter "My Soundtrack of Hope" which explains how listening to music is one of his coping mechanisms in dealing with stress and anxiety.

Thomas Kiely is a native of County Limerick. Thomas has worked up until recently for the last 16 years in a wholesale business while gaining significant experience in this role from sales, purchasing management, sourcing products and pricing specialist perspectives. This is his first published chapter in a peer reviewed publication.

Keith Russell is the creator and founder of multi award nominated mental health blog and podcast called The Endless Spiral. From an early age Keith has lived with several mental health conditions including anxiety, depression, and body dysmorphia. Keith was diagnosed with having Generalized Anxiety Disorder (GDA) and Body Dysmorphic Disorder (BDD). Following these diagnoses, Keith was inspired to create The Endless Spiral were he wanted to share his own story but also to offer both men and women a safe space to share their own personal experiences and, in turn, hopefully help erase the stigma the surrounds mental health.

Jantien Schoenmakers is a BA (Hons) Writing and Literature student at ATU Sligo. An experienced content creator and social media specialist, Jantien currently works as a Client Service Representative for one of the largest job search websites. She regularly volunteers with Rape Crisis Midwest and is an ambassador for the Hibbs Lupus Trust. This is her third time contributing as a guest author to the Mental Health For Millennials series.

About TheDocCheck.Com

Based in Athenry, Galway and Limerick, Ireland, we provide full writing consulting solutions and academic coaching for your research needs. We help you develop the individual insights you will require to achieve your optimum grade or successful proposal, grant application or business plan completion. We also specialise in content editing and document editing for the SME sector.

Our multi-disciplinary team of nine consulting staff works with individuals and groups over the age of eighteen to fully enhance your research, writing and communications portfolios. We believe in excellence, in helping you to attain the best possible grade – and we have achieved this since 2007 with consistent honours grades awarded to our clients. We work across all academic disciplines with qualitative and quantitative expertise, providing academic mentoring, one-to-one supervision for your research needs, thesis/project consulting solutions, proofreading, forensic editing and bespoke training.

Check out the many genuine reviews from real people Testimonials on our website, our Facebook Page, Instagram @DissertationDoctor or on our Twitter @ThesisClinic written by clients who have availed of, and believe in our service and have been kind enough to endorse us. Find us at www.thedoccheck.com